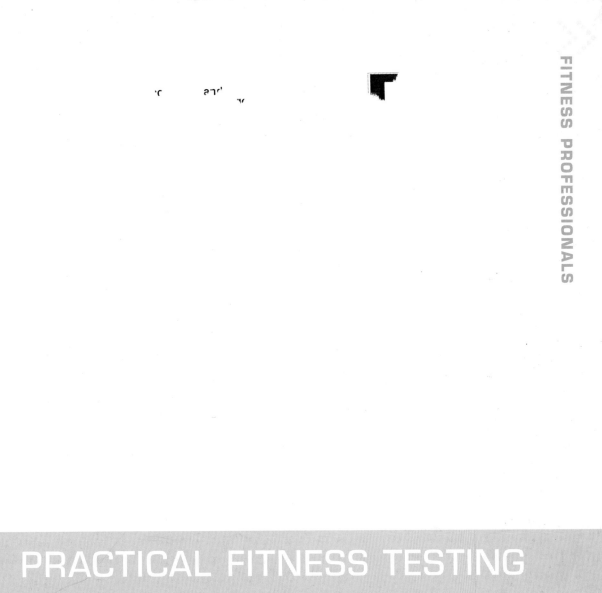

PRACTICAL FITNESS TESTING

FITNESS PROFESSIONALS

PRACTICAL FITNESS TESTING

MORC COULSON AND DAVID ARCHER

A & C BLACK · LONDON

Note

While every effort has been made to ensure that the content of this book is as technically accurate and as sound as possible, neither the authors nor the publishers can accept responsibility for any injury or loss sustained as a result of the use of this material.

Published by A&C Black Publishers Ltd
36 Soho Square, London W1D 3QY
www.acblack.com

Copyright © 2009 Morc Coulson and David Archer

ISBN 978 1 4081 1022 5

A CIP catalogue record for this book is available from the British Library.

Acknowledgements
Cover photograph © www.istockphoto.com
Inside photographs © Joanne Miller, except pp. 24–6, 126–7 Morc Coulson
Illustrations by Jeff Edwards

This book is produced using paper that is made from wood grown in managed, sustainable forests. It is natural, renewable and recyclable. The logging and manufacturing processes conform to the environmental regulations of the country of origin.

Typeset in 10.5 on 12.5pt Berthold Baskerville Regular by Palimpsest Book Production Limited, Grangemouth, Stirlingshire

Printed and bound in Spain by GraphyCems

CONTENTS

FOREWORD

'Having been a competitive athlete for many years, I understand how important fitness testing can be. Regular testing allows the athlete and the coach to check the progress of the training programme, but it also helps the athlete focus on short-term goals by providing a measure of their performance compared to their peers. I believe that there are many athletes who could benefit from regular health and fitness testing. *Practical Fitness Testing* offers a comprehensive guide to the theory and practical application of health and fitness testing for coaches and instructors of all levels across all sports and events.'

Chris Cook
Athens and Beijing Olympic Games competitor in swimming, 2004, 2008
World Championships Bronze medallist, 2006
Commonwealth Games Gold medallist, 2006
British and Commonwealth record holder in swimming

INTRODUCTION

One of the many aims of fitness testing is to collect information about the progress of an exercise programme.

When someone starts out on a training programme, they usually agree goals with their coach or instructor. Testing can both establish whether those goals have been met, and what adjustments, if any, could be made.

The entire testing process, irrespective of the methods used, can be thought of as a cyclical process as shown in figure 0.1.

This cyclical process provides the coach or

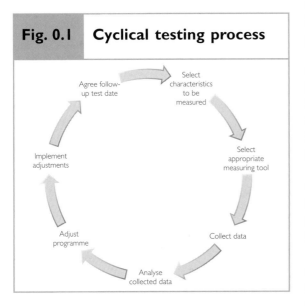

Fig. 0.1 **Cyclical testing process**

Select characteristics to be measured

Select appropriate measuring tool

Collect data

Analyse collected data

Adjust programme

Implement adjustments

Agree follow-up test date

instructor with a standardised, easy-to-follow format that can be repeated on an ongoing basis.

Once you have decided what you want to test (for example strength, aerobic capacity, flexi-

bility etc appropriate to the subject and their sport or event), you can select the method that will best measure it with the resources available. Test data can then be collected, analysed and interpreted so that adjustments to the individual's training programme can be made. Analysis of test results often becomes easier as you gain more experience but it is important that you remain objective and use the most appropriate form of analysis relevant to the subject.

The results of a one-off test provide the baseline from which to construct an appropriate exercise programme but you need to carry out further testing in order to continue to assess and progress that programme.

Practical Fitness Testing has been written as a reference guide for those regularly involved in fitness or health testing. It deals with both laboratory and field-based testing and is useful for coaches and instructors who do not have access to the particular facilities or specialist equipment required in more formal testing environments.

This book will give you a basic understanding of the principles related to health and fitness testing and the cyclical process described earlier, and suggest suitable and practical tests related to particular characteristics, events or sports.

The book describes in detail a range of health and fitness testing methods (or protocols, as they are known), and describes the methods of analysing the data and classifying the results according to published specific population data.

Within the book, tests are divided into two general categories: *health tests* and *fitness tests*. Health tests can be carried out on anyone and are used to assess readiness for undertaking exercise programmes. Fitness tests are usually carried out on people who are more active, and are used to assess the performance of particular characteristics or parameters. The following is a brief overview of each chapter.

Chapter 1 deals with the analysis and classification of specific data derived from basic test measurements, such as muscular strength, body fat percentage and lung function. The chapter also deals with the meaning and treatment of terms such as validity, accuracy, objectivity, reliability and normative data in the context of health and fitness testing. The chapter explores the difference between laboratory and field testing, direct and indirect tests, and maximal and submaximal testing, and provides examples in each related area. Sources of measurement error and variation regarding equipment and biological differences are also discussed. Finally, this chapter deals with the area of statistical analysis for the interpretation of test data. Topics such as average values, standard deviations, correlation and t-tests are all addressed.

Chapter 2 discusses the meaning of fitness in terms of both health and performance, and addresses the importance of being 'physically fit'. The chapter also describes the most commonly agreed components of fitness and discusses which of these are most important for specific sports, activities or events. It looks at energy systems and their contribution to exercise, particularly at different intensities and durations. For a more detailed description of energy systems please refer to *The Fitness Instructor's Handbook* by Morc Coulson and *The Advanced Fitness Instructor's Handbook* by Morc Coulson and David Archer, both published by A&C Black.

Chapter 3 deals with a range of health tests commonly used by coaches and instructors, and the issues of screening and informed consent.

The tests include heart rate, blood pressure and lung function. It looks at the underpinning knowledge required and the area of health it relates to. As well as an overview of each test, there is step-by-step instruction on how to administer each of the described tests. There is also explanation of how to deal with the test results from an analysis perspective. Finally, there is a classification for each test, which provides comparative data from various populations.

Chapter 4 deals with tests related to body composition, the estimation of body fat percentage and the difference between direct and indirect testing methods. This topic has been given a chapter of its own due to the amount of information available. The chapter explains the different components of body mass and describes a variety of ways to estimate them (using prediction equations). The chapter also provides instructions on how to identify landmarks on the body, and how to carry out certain body composition assessments using those landmarks.

The remaining chapters follow the same format as chapter 4 but deal with tests related to fitness or performance; all tests in these chapters are considered dynamic in nature as opposed to the health tests in chapters 3 and 4, which are often considered to be static.

Chapter 5 covers flexibility testing in comprehensive detail and introduces the terms 'static' and 'dynamic' flexibility, discussing their importance in a sports and fitness environment as well as in a health environment. Testing methodologies are described covering areas such as anatomical reference points and factors that can affect joint range of motion. Joint stability and the mechanisms of contribution are also addressed. The chapter discusses the limitations of indirect testing methods and the difficulties in testing dynamic flexibility. It also looks at interpretation, comparison and evaluation of the results of measurements of flexibility.

Chapter 6 is dedicated to tests relating to muscular strength and endurance. Various terms are explained as well as factors that determine both strength and endurance. Advantages and disadvantages of using resistance machines and free weights are discussed in detail from a testing perspective. Issues concerning maximal and sub-maximal muscular strength testing are explored in the light of the huge range of research in this area. Also from a research perspective, the issue of muscular strength being affected by age, gender, velocity of movement, joint angle and other factors is addressed.

Chapter 7 is concerned with testing speed and agility. It describes how to identify sprinting phases and typical sprint distances covered (and typical times associated with each sprint distance). It looks at what factors affect the development of speed and the contribution of stride rate and stride length. There are descriptions of standard speed and agility tests as well as how to modify tests for specific subjects or activities.

Chapter 8 deals with power testing in the context of cardiovascular or resistance exercises for sporting or athletic performance. Explanations are given of terms such as power, anaerobic power, velocity and force, to help explain the relationship between these terms in skeletal muscle. The stretch shortening cycle, and its contribution to explosive power movements, is described in detail with reference to the plethora of research carried out in this area. The origin and development of jump testing is discussed and the chapter deals with the concepts of 'oxygen debt' and 'critical power' and how they can be used to estimate anaerobic power and to predict performance.

Chapter 9 is entitled 'Aerobic endurance testing', which is essentially maximal and sub-maximal tests designed to measure VO_2 max. Factors affecting aerobic capacity are discussed, as are the differences between modes of testing. The chapter also outlines various advantages and disadvantages relating to a range of direct, indirect, field-based, laboratory-based, maximal and sub-maximal tests.

Chapter 10 deals with the extensive subjects of 'blood lactate' testing and 'anaerobic threshold' testing. The chapter explores the concept of anaerobic threshold and the link between lactate and ventilatory threshold. As this chapter deals mainly with laboratory-based testing techniques, health and safety issues are discussed in relation to blood sampling. Finally, the relationship between blood lactate and muscle lactate concentrations is explained.

Where possible, throughout this book there are references and prices for the equipment required for each particular test, to help the coach or instructor determine the potential set-up costs for administering tests. There is a reference list at the end of each chapter if you want to investigate a particular topic in more depth. You should also be aware that health and fitness testing is a scientific area that is constantly updating. Ongoing research not only helps to develop rigorous test protocols, but also provides comparative data in the form of normative values as discussed later in the book.

Testing, when carried out as accurately as possible, is a valuable tool for coaches and instructors of all levels regardless of their background or experience. It is hoped that this book can help you gain more of an interest in this area and enhance training or exercise programmes to the benefit of all concerned.

This book has also been written to help those instructors in the health and fitness industry achieve what is known as Continuing Professional Development (CPD) points. This can be done by accessing an online multiple-choice exam and, if successful, gaining CPD points that are allocated to the book and exam paper. This can also be done for two other books written by the authors:

1. Coulson, M. (2007) *Fitness Professionals: The Fitness Instructor's Handbook*, A&C Black
2. Coulson, M. & Archer, D. (2008) *Fitness Professionals: The Advanced Fitness Instructor's Handbook*, A&C Black

The details for the multiple-choice question paper and allocated CPD points are explained in the next section and also on the website www.ukcentre4fitness.co.uk.

Continuing professional development points

CPD is related to the health and fitness industry and the Register of Exercise Professionals (REPs), which is overseen by a body known as SkillsActive.

SkillsActive is licensed by government as the Sector Skills Council for Active Leisure and Learning. Directed by employers, SkillsActive leads the skills and productivity drive across the sport and recreation, health and fitness, outdoors, playwork, and caravan industries – known as the active leisure and learning sector.

SkillsActive works with health and fitness professionals across the UK to ensure the workforce is appropriately skilled and qualified. This includes working with higher and further education in developing frameworks for new qualifications so graduates can leave college or university with industry recognised vocational qualifications.

The Register of Exercise Professionals has also been set up to help safeguard and promote the health and interests of people who are using the services of exercise and fitness instructors, teachers and trainers. The Register of Exercise Professionals uses a process of self-regulation that recognises industry-based qualifications and practical competency, and requires fitness professionals to work to a Code of Ethical Practice within the framework of National Occupational Standards developed by SkillsActive. Qualifications needed to gain entry to the register are closely aligned with National Occupational Standards.

Once accepted onto the register, instructors must continue their personal development by attending a minimum number of hours each year in the format of further qualifications, workshops, seminars or conferences that have been accredited by REPs, in order to remain on the register. This is known as continuing professional development, or CPD. There are many courses, seminars, workshops and events available across the UK that are accredited for CPD points, delivered by a diverse range of organisations such as private training providers, colleges and universities. Books and journal articles can also be accredited with CPD points. The number of CPD points depends on the relationship of the course to National Occupational Standards, the number of hours of the course, if there is some form of assessment, and the learning outcomes. A full list of entry qualifications and CPD courses is available from REPs at www.exerciseregister.org.

This book has been awarded two CPD points by the Register of Exercise Professionals, so if you already hold an industry qualification you can use it as part of your professional development. If you are looking to gain an extra two CPD points you can access an online multiple-choice exam based on the information within this book at www.ukcentre4fitness.co.uk. Continuing professional development points can also be gained in the same way with the two books mentioned previously.

BASIC MEASUREMENT AND ANALYSIS

OBJECTIVES

After completing this chapter you should be able to:

1 Understand the meaning of terms such as validity, accuracy, objectivity and reliability.

2 Explain the difference between normative-referenced and criterion-referenced standards.

3 List the guidelines for pre-testing, during testing and post-testing that help to standardise testing.

4 List and describe the different types of test validity.

5 List and describe a range of terminology related to statistics.

6 Explain the difference between laboratory and field testing, direct and indirect tests, and maximal and sub-maximal testing, and provide examples of each.

7 Understand, and calculate, average values and standard deviations related to data sets.

8 Understand sources of measurement error and variation with regards to equipment and biological variability.

9 List a range of statistical functions that are available in Excel.

10 View basic statistical analysis methods such as correlation and student t-tests.

11 List a range of benefits related to health and fitness testing.

12 Explain the difference between static and dynamic tests and give an example of each.

Self-study task

You are just starting to work as a freelance personal trainer and one of the products you offer in a client's fitness assessment is a body fat percentage check (see chapter 4 for further details).

In your business plan, you allocated a maximum of £1500 for body composition equipment. The options available are:

- Bodystat 1500, a device that measures single frequency bioimpedance (the response of a living organism to an externally applied electric current) and uses this to assess body fat percentage. £500 www.bodystat.com
- Bodystat QuadScan, a device that measures multi-frequency bioimpedance and uses this to assess body fat percentage. £2000 www.bodystat.com
- Harpenden skinfold callipers. Textbook of kinanthropometry £200
- Harpenden skinfold callipers. Textbook of kinanthropometry, two-day course in anthropometry provided by ISAK (International Society of Applied Kinanthropometry) £1200

Task

Go to the web links and find information about how well you can reproduce measurements using the equipment. Think about how you would justify your choice of body composition equipment.

Testing terminology

There is a great deal of specific terminology used in a range of literature (both scientific and non-scientific) relating to fitness and health testing. Some of the most commonly used terminology used is explained below:

Subject

This simply refers to the individual that is undertaking the test.

Test

Test is synonymous with the term *measurement*. For instance, a measurement of strength is the same as a test of strength.

Evaluation

This is a statement about the quality or value of what has been assessed and thus involves the tester making a decision, so interpreting a score. For example, is a one repetition max (1RM) bench press of 50kg good for a 55-year-old, 70kg body mass, untrained man?

Standards (normative- and criterion-referenced)

To make an evaluation of a test, there needs to be something to compare it against. The test must be referenced to some standards, which should be as relevant as possible to the subject in terms of gender, age and body mass. For many exercise- and health-related measures this is performed by comparing the values obtained to *norm-referenced standards* (otherwise known as normative or norm values), which have been gained from test scores of other subjects. So, for the 55-year-old, 70kg body mass, untrained man mentioned above, the classification can be checked. For example, did he fit into the classification of 'poor', 'fair', 'average' or 'superior'? In other cases, the performance may be assessed relative to a criterion that is set for them, either by the tester or by a governing body/health executive. One example of this is the concept of Body Mass Index (BMI), which will be introduced in chapter 4. The subject's BMI could be assessed relative to the criterion for underweight, overweight or obese individuals (18.5, 25 and 30 respectively).

Reliability/reproducibility

The reliability of a test simply refers to how reproducible the test is. For example, if the same test is repeated (without any change in status of the person being tested) and similar results are obtained, then the test can be said to be reliable. Also known as reproducibility, reliability refers to the amount of variation that occurs in the test results between repeated trials. Essentially there are two main sources of potential variation that can affect the reliability of the test, those of *biological variation* and *experimental error*.

Biological variation

When any measurements on a living creature are made, there is a certain natural variation. Something seemingly as constant as height changes slightly from day to day and typically varies by 1cm during the day! Body mass typically varies by 0.2–0.5 per cent from day to day and a measurement such as heart rate (HR) in beats per minute (bpm) typically varies by much more. Running at 10mph (16km/h) on a treadmill could elicit an average HR of 178bpm one day and 180bpm the following day solely due to biological variation. An awareness of the magnitude of this biological variation is vital, as a subject's exercising HR at a fixed workload of 178 one day and 190 on the following day may indicate something is wrong, such as dehydration or overtraining.

Experimental error

Experimental error can be associated with the testing environment, equipment used and the error of the tester/assessor. Tester error mainly depends on the tester's experience and the complexity of the test. Correct training and practice can reduce this kind of error. For example, the use of skinfold callipers involves identifying the correct anatomical sites, lifting the correct thickness of skinfold and reading the dial at the correct angle. This may take the tester thousands of measurements until the technique is developed sufficiently to reduce error to an acceptable amount.

An indication of the testing errors can be obtained through the measurement of a statistical term called the *coefficient of variation* (described later in this chapter). At the other extreme, for a simple task, e.g. when measuring body mass using digital scales, the tester is simply recording the values obtained and the potential errors involved are reduced. In this case, the most important action for the tester is to ensure that a proper protocol is followed, e.g. for consistency, the subject is not wearing shoes/trainers, scales are *tared* (zeroed) before use, subject is fasted (if required) etc. Due to the greater error involved, skinfold thickness is typically measured in triplicate for each site, whereas body mass is typically measured only once.

In relation to equipment error, when performing expired gas analysis, which is vital in many performance- and health-related measures, the analysers used have a measurement error of approximately 1–2 per cent in terms of gas volumes and 0.1 per cent in terms of oxygen and carbon dioxide concentration. This results in certain errors in measurement of 1–3

per cent, even when working properly, due to the limitations of the procedure.

An important aspect of minimising experimental error is to ensure that all the equipment used in testing is properly calibrated before use. This should be performed regularly with a known standard depending on the accuracy or reliability required for the test. One example of poor practice known to the authors is the use of a faulty linear transducer (see chapter 8) to measure speed, power and velocity during resistance training in a group of Olympic medal winning field-eventers. The cable attached to the transducer was broken and subsequently repaired and used for another season. However, when compared to a new transducer, the measurements were nearly 50 per cent different from the correct values and thus would have resulted in incorrect assessment of speed, power and velocity and possibly errors in prescribing training intensities. Some equipment is easier to calibrate than others, but using uncalibrated equipment can lead to serious errors.

When conducting any type of test (whether field or laboratory based as explained later), an attempt should be made to keep the testing or experimental error to a minimum. One way is by standardising the test procedures (or protocol) of the test to be carried out. The following guidelines relating to the test environment will help the tester to reduce the risk of errors and improve the reliability of tests being carried out. Those involved in testing should try to implement these guidelines each time they perform fitness or health tests.

- Standardise the measuring techniques used.
- Standardise the testing environment, temperature (between 18 and 23°C) and humidity (less than 70 per cent) of an indoor testing environment. Ensure good ventilation.
- Take repeat measures at the same time of day as the original test.

- Follow a consistent procedure, i.e. number of subjects tested at a time, the presence or absence of observers, the amount of motivation given by observers, the sequence of the tests and the amount of rest time between tests.
- Standardise the amount of warm-up and practice allowed by all subjects.
- Record precise details of the test protocol (method) and measuring techniques used for future repeatability.
- During the test, standardise motivation and instructions.
- Ensure that the testing environment has immediate access to first-aid facilities and has a first-aid qualified person on hand.
- Ensure that telephone numbers and addresses of hospitals and doctors are listed and placed by the telephone in the testing environment.
- Pre-test, during-test and post-test procedures are as important as environmental guidelines for reducing the risk of experimental error. In order to help reduce this risk of error, those involved in testing should try to follow the guidelines in table 1.1 before, during and after each test or series of tests that is carried out.

Table 1.1	Pre-, during- and post-test guidelines
Procedures	Guidelines
Pre-test	• Ensure in the days leading up to testing that subjects have the opportunity to become familiar with testing procedures and any equipment that will be used. • Make sure all assistants involved are fully briefed in advance of the test. • Obtain the subject's informed consent and ensure that they receive medical clearance (where appropriate) prior to any testing. • Ensure all subjects are fully screened. • Standardise the pre-test conditions. • Ensure that subjects follow a normal diet in the days leading up to physiological assessment and also ensure that subjects do not eat two hours prior to the test (water is allowed unless the test specifies not).
During-test	• Encouragement and motivation should be standardised during the test. • On a test day subjects should be advised to avoid smoking, drinking alcohol, tea or coffee, and any similar substances. • All subjects should be advised to wear appropriate clothing for the test (let them know in advance). • The test procedure and objectives should be fully explained to all involved in the testing. • Ensure that all subjects should be free from illness and injury on the day of the testing.
Post-test	• Check the test in terms of compliance. • Check data collection for accuracy. • Organise subject feedback.

Validity

When choosing a fitness or health test it is important that it is specifically designed to measure what the tester is investigating. For example, the sit-and-reach test is not designed to measure shoulder flexibility (it is a measure of back and hamstring flexibility and is therefore considered not to be a valid test for shoulder flexibility). In other words, the validity of a particular test indicates the extent to which a test measures what it originally intended to measure.

Validity can be defined in a number of ways but, for the purpose of this book, the following will be used for explanation:

'The degree to which a test or instrument measures what it purports to measure can be categorised as logical, content, criterion, or construct validity.'
(Thomas and Nelson, 2001)

In theory, the measure of the validity of a test can be determined by comparing the results of the test with the results of another test that is known to be a valid measure of the characteristic being investigated. The most valid testing method for any characteristic is known as the *criterion measure* or sometimes the *gold standard.* There are three ways that are often used to determine whether a test measures what it is supposed to measure from a validity perspective: these are *content, criterion* and *construct validity* as are described in table 1.2.

Finally, for a test to be considered valid, it must be both reliable and relevant as explained previously. It is quite common that most tests are either one or the other but usually not both. For example, an individual's body mass index measurement is easy to perform (only height and weight required) and quite reproducible from day to day, but it is not considered to be a valid measure of total body fatness.

Objectivity

This is simply the degree to which multiple scorers or testers agree on the magnitude and outcome of the score or measurement being taken. A clearly defined scoring or measurement system can obviously enhance the test objectivity. However, if a number of scorers are used for a particular test and one scorer is more lenient than the others, this could create an unfair advantage and a disparity in scores. Experienced scorers can help eliminate or at least reduce this problem.

Table 1.2	Content, criterion and construct validity descriptions
Validity	Description
Content	This indicates that the test seems to be good or valid, based on logic, expert testimony and widespread use.
Criterion	This involves having an externally valid criterion for the test, e.g. hydrostatic weighing is a criterion measure for validating skinfold assessment of body fatness.
Construct	This is provided by showing that a test responds in the way one would expect, based on theoretical understanding of that characteristic.

Sensitivity

The sensitivity of a test is normally described as the degree to which the measures taken reflect an improvement in either performance or health. Sensitivity is very much related to the reproducibility of the test, the population or subjects measured, as well as several other factors. For example, an improvement in VO_2 max is often a good indication of improvement in aerobic fitness in untrained or recreationally active individuals. However, many scientists and coaches question the effectiveness of this type of indication in elite endurance athletes.

Specificity

One of the major challenges that most testers face (when testing athletes in particular) is to try to make the assessments mimic as closely as possible the activities related to the subject being tested. The following are generally reported to be the main factors to be considered when selecting or designing test protocols for specific subjects.

TEST PROTOCOL CONSIDERATIONS

- Muscle groups, type of activity and range of motion
- Intensity and duration of activity
- Energy systems recruited
- Resistive forces encountered

An example of specific test selection would be where the performance of a rower required physiological testing: it would be more appropriate to use a rowing ergometer than a treadmill.

For some subject groups, certain field-based tests may be more appropriate than laboratory-based tests.

For a subject group being tested for more health-related measures, such as aerobic fitness, a cycle ergometer or treadmill would be more appropriate.

Statistical terminology

The terms *measurement* and *statistics* should not be used interchangeably as they have different meanings. As mentioned previously, the term measurement relates to the process of obtaining a test score whereas the term statistics relates to the process of analysing that score.

If a set of test scores (data set) is just described then this is termed *descriptive statistics* as opposed to *analytical statistics* in which a relevant statistical analysis package is used to evaluate the data set.

There is a great deal of terminology related to this area and the following is a selection of the more common terms used.

Precision

The concept of precision is linked to the accuracy of the measurement taken. For example, a 30m sprint should be measured to the nearest hundredth of a second (0.01sec) and *not* to the nearest second. In another example, heart rate monitors record only to the nearest beat per minute so an averaged heart rate of 167.5bpm should be correctly recorded as 168bpm. In relation to precision and data collected, the following are terms you should understand.

Mean

The mean, or arithmetic average, is the sum of the scores divided by the number of scores.

Median

Order the numbers from low to high and the middle one, or 50th percentile, is the median.

Mode

The most frequently observed score. It is not typically a useful indicator of the average value for a measurement.

Range

The range is the maximum score minus the minimum score. It gives a measure of the variability of the data.

Standard deviation

To understand the concept of standard deviation it is useful to understand the *normal distribution* of data values. A normal distribution of data (measurements collected from a test) indicates that most of the examples in a set of data are close to the average, while relatively few examples tend to one extreme or the other. For example, a normally distributed data set plotted on a graph would have a bell-shaped appearance such as that in figure 1.1.

When transferring data (not just test data) to a graph, the x-axis (the horizontal one) represents the value of the measurement in question and the y-axis (the vertical one) is the number of data points for each value on the x-axis. Not all sets of data will have graphs that look like the one in figure 1.1, as some graphs will have relatively flat curves while other graphs will be quite steep.

The *standard deviation* as it is known is a statistic that shows how the data points are clustered around the mean (average) in a set of data. When the data points are tightly bunched together and the bell-shaped curve is steep, the standard deviation is considered to be small. When the data points are spread apart and the bell curve is relatively flat, this indicates that there is a relatively large standard deviation.

As can be seen in figure 1.2 one standard deviation away from the mean in either direction on the horizontal axis accounts for somewhere around 68 per cent of the data in the group. Two standard deviations away from the mean in either direction can account for roughly 95 per cent of the data in the group, and three standard deviations in either direction can account for about 99 per cent of the data in the group. If this bell-shaped curve were flatter and more spread out, the standard deviation would have to be larger in order to account for the respective percentages of the data. In other

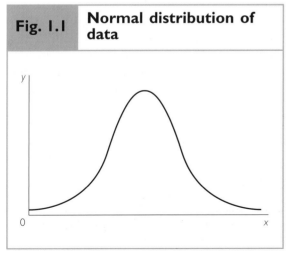

Fig. 1.1   **Normal distribution of data**

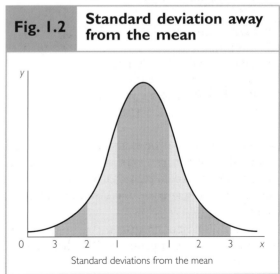

Fig. 1.2   **Standard deviation away from the mean**

Standard deviations from the mean

words, the standard deviation can show you how spread out the examples in a set of data are from the mean.

In most cases biological test data tends to be normally distributed; however, this can differ in a few cases. In cases where the data is skewed (where the bell-shaped curve moves away from the mean) to the right or skewed to the left, median and range (as defined earlier) are considered to be better ways of describing the test data.

Fig. 1.3	**Equation to calculate standard deviation**

$$\sigma = \sqrt{\frac{\sum(x - \bar{x})^2}{n - 1}}$$

- Step 1. Find the mean (average) of all the values denoted by the '$\bar{x}$' (each individual value is denoted by 'x').
- Step 2. For each value x, subtract the overall average ($\bar{x}$) from x, then multiply that result by itself (otherwise known as determining the square of that value).
- Step 3. Sum (denoted by $\sum$) all the squared values. Then divide that result by (n-1) where 'n' is the number of data values.
- Step 4. Then find the square root of that last number.

If all of the above steps are followed correctly then this gives the standard deviation (denoted in lower case by the Greek symbol σ) of a set of data values that have been collected from a particular test. If only a sample of the data set was used for analysis then the standard deviation would be denoted by the letter 's'.

Calculating standard deviation

Calculators and computers are capable of calculating standard deviation as they have in-built equations to deal with this. However, standard deviation can also be calculated by hand by following the steps in figure 1.3.

Coefficient of variation

The term *coefficient of variation* (CV) is just another term used to give an indication of the standard deviation as a percentage of the mean value. As well as knowing the standard deviation, the coefficient of variation gives you an additional tool, which can be useful when making comparisons between different groups of subjects or between different protocols used to test those subjects.

The example in table 1.3 shows the final results of squat values (measured in kilograms) taken from a female high-school volleyball team's maximal squat test measurements. The average squat of the team has already been calculated at 59kg (total of all squats divided by the number of squats) and the standard deviation has been calculated at 11kg. Dividing the standard deviation (11) by the average squat (59) and multiplying by 100 gives a coefficient of variation of 19 per cent.

Alternatively, the use of statistical analysis packages such as SPSS (statistical analysis package for social sciences), or a spreadsheet such as Excel, can quickly provide simple statistical information relating to the data collected from the test carried out. Table 1.4 gives an overview of the functions that are available within the Excel computer package.

SPSS has a much wider range of statistical tests and tools, though many basic tests can be performed using Excel or a freely available equivalent to it (www.openoffice.org). When feeding back the analysis of the data to squads or clients, Excel can be used to provide useful tables and charts of progress, targets and weaknesses. It can be a very good motivational tool when working with both teams and individuals to provide incentive and encouragement.

Table 1.3	Pre-season values of 1RM squat from female volleyball players
1RM squat (kg)	38, 45, 55, 55, 55, 60, 60, 65, 70, 72, 75
Mean	(38+45+55+55+55+60+60+65+70+72+75) / 11 = 59kg
Median	60
Mode	55
Range	75 − 38 = 37
Std deviation	11
Coefficient of variation	(11/59) × 100% = 19%

Table 1.4	Simple statistical functions in Excel
Function	Description
Average (data)	Calculates mean value ($\bar{x}$) for the data selected
Max (data)	Returns the largest value in the field selected
Min (data)	Returns the smallest value in the field selected
STDEV (data)	Calculates standard deviation for the data selected
Correl (array1, array2)	Calculates the correlation coefficient between two sets of measurements (array1 and array2 refer to the two sets of measurements selected in Excel), e.g. what is the association between 1RM squat and 20m sprint speed?
T-test (array1, array2, tails, type)	A simple statistical test (t-test) and returns the probability associated with that test (P value). It compares the means of array1 and array2. If the P value is less than 0.05, then the two are statistically different (P<0.05). Number of tails refers to whether or not you are performing a one-tailed or two-tailed test. In most cases, we use a two-tailed test, unless we are expecting only an increase or a decrease in the parameter measured. Type refers to paired or unpaired. If the measurements are made on the same individuals then you would use a paired test (1). If the measurements are on a different group of individuals, e.g. comparing the speed of the youth team to the senior team, then you would perform an unpaired test (2).

Basic statistics

You may ask: *'Why do I need to know anything about statistics such as biological variation? All I need to know is by how much each of my subjects' speed has increased and if I'm interested in the team measures, I'll just average it out.'* This would seem to be a valid opinion, but using two examples from a performance and health perspective should help demonstrate the usefulness of statistics for analysis purposes, and how potential error can at least be addressed.

There are many other occasions when understanding concepts such as validity, accuracy and precision can be vital. Different testing protocols can have different measurement errors and it may not be possible to use the most accurate and reproducible tests due to time, space or financial constraints. In these cases, we can choose the most practical option as long as we understand the limitations of the tests we undertake.

Example 1: Imagine you are managing an exercise programme with a group of clients who have been diagnosed by their GPs with high blood pressure. As part of the initial consultation you recommend the group increase its physical activity levels. You then design a training programme to help them achieve this increase in activity levels. A bout of initial baseline testing indicates an average (of the group) systolic blood pressure of 150mmHg. After two months of training, you then carry out a re-test on the group and find that their average systolic blood pressure has decreased to 147mmHg. Only by understanding the natural variation in resting blood pressure measurements can you determine if the 3mmHg change in blood pressure is sufficient to have any health effects.

Example 2: Using an online gas analyser, you carry out a test protocol on a female distance runner for the purpose of measuring her VO_2 max at the start of a training block (set period of training). The results indicate that her VO_2 max is 64ml^{-1}.kg^{-1}.min^{-1}. Following an endurance training block, you test her again and find that her VO_2 max has increased to 66ml^{-1}.kg^{-1}.min^{-1}. Does that definitely indicate that her VO_2 max has improved? Not necessarily, as the biological variation in VO_2 max is considered to be 1% and the experimental error in some cases can be as high as 3% (gas volumes using an online gas analyser are typically only within 2% of the true value). Therefore, this 3.1% 'increase' in VO_2 max could be due to variations in measurement rather than a true increase.

Correlation and prediction

The term *correlation* (or, as it is known in measurement, correlation coefficient or 'R'), describes the relationship between two measurements or groups of measurements. The result can be either a positive relationship or a negative relationship. For example, figure 1.4 shows the analysis of the relationship between measurements of 1RM squat strength and measurements of 30m sprint times. The values of 'R' can range between minus one (-1), known as a negative relationship, and plus one (+1), known as a positive relationship. The closer 'R' is either to +1 or -1, the stronger the association or relationship is. The value of R^2 can also be used as indication of the relationship and in the example in figure 1.4, R^2 is 0.9221. In this particular example it is an indication that 92 per cent of the variation in 30m sprint time can be explained by the 1RM squat. This type of analysis also allows the prediction (known as linear regression) of performance, in this case an athlete's 30m sprint time, based on their squat performance.

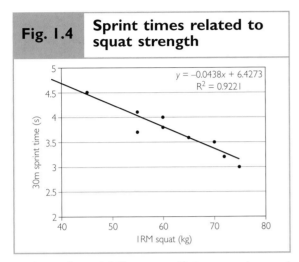

Fig. 1.4 Sprint times related to squat strength

$y = -0.0438x + 6.4273$
$R^2 = 0.9221$

A number of different coefficients can be used depending on the situation or context of the measurements to be correlated. The most common correlations in fitness and health testing tend to be the *Pearson's product-moment correlation* and the *Spearman's correlation*. Remember, however, that a correlation can only *indicate* a possible relationship between variables or groups of measurements, but does not actually confirm or establish a causal relationship. In other words, it cannot state exactly that one of the groups of measurements has a direct effect on the other group of measurements. Once a correlation has shown a possible relationship, further statistical analysis would be required to investigate the nature of the relationship.

Tests

The statistical test known as a *t-test* is most frequently used to test (the null hypothesis) that the means of two normally distributed populations are equal.

The use of a t-test is illustrated by using the data obtained on the female high school volleyball players in table 1.5. A t-test can provide a statistical indication about whether their squat values improved. Performing a t-test can be done using SPSS or Excel.

In the first instance, let us compare the squat performance of team A between year 1 and year 2. Since the data is on the same group of athletes, then a paired t-test is used and this shows that the 'P' value obtained was 0.006. As this is less than 0.05 (the usual threshold chosen for statistical significance), it shows that the squat performance for team A was significantly greater in the second year than the first (if the 'P' value was above 0.05 this would show that team A's squat performance was not significantly greater).

If we were to compare team A in season 1 to an opposing team (B), we would have to perform an 'unpaired' t-test (independent t-test) as we are comparing two different groups. The result of the unpaired t-test shows that the 'P' value obtained was 0.34. As this is greater than 0.05, it shows that there is no significant difference in performance between the two teams.

Paired t-tests are more powerful than unpaired

Table 1.5	Squat performance for female volleyball teams A and B			
	Team A Year 1	Team A Year 2	Team B Year 1	Team A Year 3
Mean	59kg	62kg	58kg	62kg
Standard deviation	11kg	12kg	11kg	12kg
P value (relative to Team A, Year 1)		0.006 (<0.05)	0.34 (>0.05)	0.001 (<0.05)
P value (relative to Team A, Year 2)				0.92 (>0.05)

t-tests, as there is less variability in the results because the same subjects are being tested.

One-way ANOVA

If we were to follow up the team for another season, to continue to track their progress we would have another set of statistics to analyse. Even though t-tests are simple to perform, they should only be used when comparing two sets of data. In the case of year 3, we must perform what is called a one-way analysis of variance (ANOVA).

The factor we are investigating in our current test is called time: have they improved over time? Performing a one-way ANOVA using SPSS with the data provided indicates that there was a significant difference between the groups. However, a further analysis known as a 'post-hoc' test is required to see whether they improved from year to year.

Two-way ANOVA could be used if we were looking at more than one factor: for example, if we wanted to break down the volleyball players into offensive and defensive positions to see if both groups got stronger over the three years. These two-way ANOVA and post-hoc tests are beyond the scope of this book and readers are advised to read a text such as Thomas and Nelson (2001) for further details.

Health and fitness testing

One of the many objectives of health and fitness testing is to establish a comprehensive physiological profile of an individual. If fitness levels are established as a result of testing, a more detailed and accurate exercise programme can

Table 1.6	Benefits of fitness testing
Benefit of testing	Description of benefit
Identify strengths and weaknesses	Testing can help to establish an overall picture of the individual's physical condition. It also provides baseline data for training programmes and can help to assess an individual's health status, acting as a monitor for over-training.
Monitor progress	By repeating tests at specific intervals, the effectiveness of the current training programme can be monitored. Results also provide a useful motivational tool to encourage individuals.
Grouping	Testing can provide information to group individuals according to ability.
Education	Testing can help to provide a better understanding of the demands of the particular sport or event.
Recovery guide	Testing is a useful way to assess recovery from injury and readiness for training.
Motivation	Testing can be used to set standards and motivate subjects.
Goal setting	Short- and long-term objectives can be established.

be designed with a view to re-testing following a sufficiently long period of training.

This book is concerned with testing where there is limited access to a variety of testing equipment. For a more clinically based explanation of test protocols, you should access the recommended reading stated at the end of each chapter.

Health and fitness testing can be of benefit to the coach, instructor and subject in many ways as can be seen in table 1.6.

There are many situations in which health and fitness testing can take place. It is important that you are aware of the range and diversity of these situations.

Laboratory and field tests

Testing can take place either in a laboratory environment (see figure 1.5a), which usually involves the use of expensive and technical equipment, or in a field-based environment (see figure 1.5b) in which the test can be taken to the subject and is often less expensive. For decades, laboratory tests have generally been found to be more accurate, but in recent years certain field tests have become comparable to laboratory versions.

Direct and indirect testing

In many cases testing measures directly what is being investigated, known as *direct testing*. The simplest example of a direct test is a standard laboratory-based VO_2 max test (see chapter 9). In this test, measurements of the maximal volume of oxygen consumed during the test, directly through the collection of expired gases, is carried out.

Alternatively, an example of an indirect test of VO_2 max would be the multi-stage fitness test or the Cooper 12-minute run test (chapter 9). In these particular tests there is a measure, such as a stage number or a distance run, that is used to estimate or predict VO_2 max (these predictions are based on statistical relationships obtained in a laboratory environment).

Direct tests, unfortunately, are often impractical or impossible to carry out. For example, it would not be feasible to carry out a direct body fat test, as all the fat from the individual

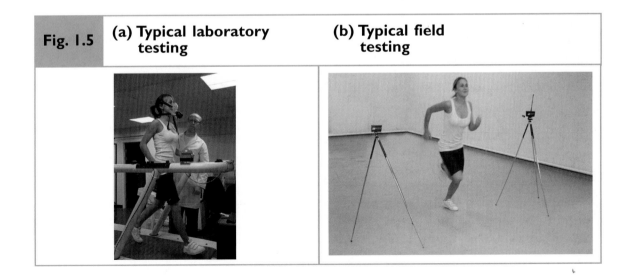

Fig. 1.5   **(a) Typical laboratory testing**   **(b) Typical field testing**

being tested would have to be removed, which might be quite painful!

Maximal and sub-maximal testing

The decision to use maximal or sub-maximal tests depends largely on the requirements for the data, the subject being tested, and the aims or reasons for the test being carried out. Maximal testing, as the term implies, has the disadvantage of requiring exercise to volitional fatigue. This type of testing may even, in some cases, require the supervision of a physician and emergency equipment. Sub-maximal testing just refers to tests that do not require the subject to go to maximal fatigue.

Static and dynamic tests

Even though the number of available health and fitness tests is extensive, tests can be broadly categorised into two groups known as static tests and dynamic tests. With static tests there is no form of exercise required. With dynamic tests some form of exercise or exertion must be carried out. Table 1.7 shows a range of typical static and dynamic tests used for both health and performance purposes.

One of the many concerns is the order of the tests to be carried out if more than one test (normally referred to as a test battery) is to be

performed. The order of the testing and the recovery times between each test must be care-

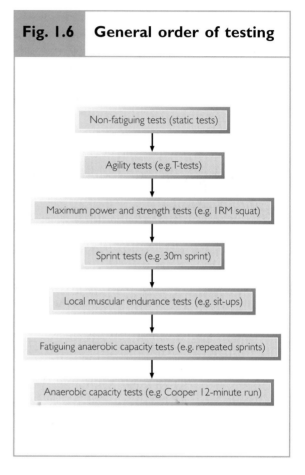

Fig. 1.6   General order of testing

Non-fatiguing tests (static tests)

↓

Agility tests (e.g. T-tests)

↓

Maximum power and strength tests (e.g. 1RM squat)

↓

Sprint tests (e.g. 30m sprint)

↓

Local muscular endurance tests (e.g. sit-ups)

↓

Fatiguing anaerobic capacity tests (e.g. repeated sprints)

↓

Anaerobic capacity tests (e.g. Cooper 12-minute run)

Table 1.7	Typical static and dynamic tests
	Typical tests
Static tests	Heart rate, blood pressure, lung function (peak expiratory flow, forced vital capacity), anthropometric measurements (height, weight, body fat %), sit and reach.
Dynamic tests	Muscular strength, muscular endurance, power, speed, VO_2 max, lactate threshold.

fully thought through as these can depend largely on the specific energy systems recruited during the chosen tests. Even though there is no specific testing order suitable for all multiple test procedures, the general order of testing shown in figure 1.6 on p. 14 could be as used (Baechle and Earle 2000).

Irrespective of the type of tests being carried out, it is a useful procedure when carrying out multiple tests to record the results using some form of standardised recording mechanism. This testing record should be kept for future reference but as it would normally contain confidential information, it should be kept in a secure place.

The date of the testing procedure should always be recorded so that each test record can be used to compare against subsequent tests. This is extremely useful as it can be used to justify any programme adjustment or alteration decisions.

Although there are many health and fitness testing score sheets available in books or on the Internet (or you could design your own), table 1.8 is an example of a typical score sheet commonly used by coaches and instructors.

Table 1.8	Example fitness testing score sheet				
Test	Score	Category	Test	Score	Category	Comments
Blood pressure	Syst._____ Dias._____		Standing broad jump	m_____		
Peak flow			Vertical jump	cm_____		
Body fat %	mm_____ %_____		Walk test	Time_____ VO_2_____		
Sit and reach	cm_____		Step test	bpm_____ VO_2_____		
Curl-up			MSFT	Level_____ VO_2_____		
Press-up			Cooper 12 min	m_____ VO_2_____		
Grip strength			Agility			
1RM	Chest_____ Leg_____					

Further reading

Baumgartner, T. A., Strong, C. H. & Hensley, L. D. (2002) *Conducting and Reading Research in Health and Human Performance*, Berkshire, UK: McGraw Hill

Blaxter, L., Hughes, C. & Tight, M. (1996) *How to Research*, Buckingham, UK: Open University Press

Bowling, A. (2002) *Research Methods in Health: Investigating health and health services*, 2nd edn, Buckingham, UK: Open University Press

Brace, N., Kemp, R. and Snelgar, R. (2006) 'SPSS for Psychologists'. *A Guide to Data Analysis Using SPSS for Windows*, 3rd edn, London: Palgrave

Gratton, C. & Jones, I. (2004) *Research Methods for Sport Studies*, London, UK: Routledge

Graziano, A. & Raulin, M. (2003) *Research Methods: A process of inquiry*, 5th edn, Boston, Massachusetts: Pearson

Kinnear, P. & Gray, C. (1999) *SPSS for Windows Made Simple*, Hove, UK: Psychology Press

Northedge, A., Thomas, J., Lane, A. & Peasgood, A. (1997) *The Sciences Good Study Guide*, Milton Keynes, UK: Open University Press

Pallant, J. (2001) *SPSS Survival Manual: A step-by-step guide to data analysis using SPSS for Windows (Version 10 and 11)*, Maidenhead, UK: Open University Press

Safrit, J. M. & Wood, M. T. (1995) *Introduction to Measurement in Physical Education and Exercise Science*, 3rd edn, St. Louis, Missouri: Mosby

Thomas, J. R. & Nelson, J. K. (2001) *Research Methods in Physical Activity*, 4th edn, Champaign, Illinois: Human Kinetics

WHAT IS FITNESS?

2

OBJECTIVES

After completing this chapter you should be able to:

1　Understand the meaning of fitness in terms of health and performance.

2　List and describe the components of fitness.

3　Describe the term 'aerobic capacity' and state the units used to measure it.

4　Assess which components of fitness are most important for specific sports or activities.

5　State the difference between muscular strength and muscular endurance.

6　Explain what is meant by the term 'power' and its components in the context of fitness training.

7　Simply define the terms 'speed' and 'agility'.

8　Explain what is meant by the term 'body composition'.

9　Define the term 'flexibility' and list the different types of stretches that can be used to improve it.

10　Recognise the importance of physical fitness in terms of health and disease.

11　List and describe the various components of fitness required for sports such as team sports, endurance events, speed events, and strength and power sports.

12　Understand the energy systems and their contribution to exercise of different intensities and durations.

Components of fitness

The common term *fitness*, which is often used wrongly in a sporting or health and fitness environment, can be a difficult construct or concept to define simply. Fitness, or the term *fit for purpose*, could relate to performance at a competitive level or just to performance of everyday tasks from a health perspective. Fitness, therefore, can be related to either performance or health.

In relation to health, the requirements of fitness would be different from the requirements for performance, as it would focus on lifestyle issues and keeping the body free of disease. For the purpose of this book, however, the focus will be on fitness for performance (even though health will be covered briefly), which is sometimes referred to as *physical fitness*.

Physical fitness, as with fitness for health, is not considered to be a single construct as it can be divided into several discrete components that can be trained or adapted individually. The emphasis placed on training each component of fitness would depend on the nature of the sport or event that the individual is training for. Depending on the source or author, these discrete physical fitness components vary but often include areas such as *aerobic endurance, anaerobic threshold, muscular strength and endurance, power, speed and agility, body composition* and *flexibility* as can be seen in figure 2.1.

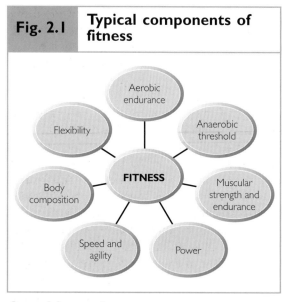

Fig. 2.1 Typical components of fitness

Aerobic endurance

Aerobic endurance is sometimes known as *aerobic capacity*, which, in simple terms, refers to the ability of the heart, lungs and associated vessels to deliver oxygen to the working muscles (and subsequently for the muscles to use this oxygen to generate work output).

Aerobic endurance is normally measured as *volume of oxygen (VO$_2$)* with VO$_2$ max being defined as *the maximum amount of oxygen that can be delivered to and utilised by the working muscles*. The units that are used to measure VO$_2$ are millilitres of oxygen for each kilogram of bodyweight used up every minute, which is written as $mlO_2.kg^{-1}min^{-1}$. This can be described as the amount of oxygen delivered to each kilogram of the body each minute. In absolute terms this can also be measured in litres of oxygen per minute ($l.min^{-1}$). Training for aerobic endurance can be done with little or no equipment and take many forms.

Improvements in aerobic endurance typically occur when the exercise involves using large muscle groups over a prolonged period of time, at an intensity (work rate) that would be classed as aerobic (walking, hiking, running, stepping, swimming, cycling, dancing, skiing, skipping etc, while the participant can still maintain a conversation). Anaerobic levels involve participants exercising at higher intensities.

Even though there are many fitness benefits associated with aerobic exercise, there are also many health benefits (covered later in this chapter). One of the most important commonly cited health benefits of undertaking a programme of aerobic-type exercise is that of a reduced risk of contracting some form of Coronary Artery Disease (CAD). Other benefits include the following:

- Reduced blood pressure
- Reduced body fat
- Reduced blood lipids (fats)
- Lowered heart rate for a given intensity of exercise
- Increased exercise threshold for accumulation of blood lactate
- Increased capillarisation
- Increased ability to deliver oxygen to the working muscles
- Increase in HDL (good) cholesterol
- Increase in self-esteem and global self-worth

For the coach or participant, there are many ways to test aerobic endurance depending on the sporting context. As far as being a component of fitness, aerobic endurance is usually considered to be an important, integral part of a training programme for most sports or events and is therefore often tested for the purpose of measuring and monitoring improvement. There are many tests that can be administered for the purpose of measuring aerobic endurance, however, and the range of tests will be covered later in this book.

Anaerobic threshold

The term *anaerobic threshold* is the point at which the energy required by the exercise can no longer be met by the aerobic system, so the anaerobic system needs to contribute substantially.

Exercising at aerobic levels is explained later in this chapter; however, exercising at intensity levels approaching 100 per cent VO_2 max or above can be referred to as anaerobic-type training. This can also be described as exercise performed at a level where the supply of energy, in the form of adenosine triphosphate (ATP), comes predominantly from systems that do not use oxygen in the stages of breakdown, i.e. ATP-PC (phosphagen) and anaerobic glycolysis, as described later in this chapter.

Anaerobic training has several sub-components such as resistance training, power training, endurance training and sprint training. A component of endurance training is speed endurance (or anaerobic endurance as it is sometimes called), and this can again be divided into short-term or long-term depending on the energy systems targeted (ATP-PC and anaerobic glycolysis). *Short-term anaerobic endurance training* increases the ability to perform maximal work for a short period of time, and *long-term anaerobic endurance training* improves the ability to maintain exercise at a high intensity.

Unlike adaptations to aerobic endurance training (see chapter 9), adaptations to anaerobic training mainly occur in the muscle groups used in the exercise. For example, in order to recruit fast-twitch type II muscle fibres (see chapter 6), the exercise intensity must be high (anaerobic). There is, however, still a role for the aerobic system as recovery from high-intensity exercise is increased, especially with a well-developed aerobic system (which can be important when performing repeated bouts of intense efforts as in team sports).

Exercise repetitions performed on a regular basis at speeds of 100 per cent VO_2 max (velocity of VO_2 max) are often very effective in improving VO_2 max and running economy,

since they are more aerobic in nature and more repetitions can be performed than in anaerobic training (for a more detailed explanation please refer to *The Advanced Fitness Instructor's Handbook* (Coulson and Archer 2008)). This demonstrates that anaerobic training can result in some training of the aerobic system if the exercise durations or repetitions are long enough.

It should also be pointed out that, in order to increase the level of the anaerobic threshold (the exercise intensity at which the contribution of anaerobic sources of energy substantially increases), aerobic training is essential.

If the aerobic system can be trained to its maximum potential then this would delay the point at which the anaerobic system would be required. In other words, anaerobic threshold is greatly influenced by the capacity of the aerobic system.

Determination of anaerobic threshold is often carried out in laboratory environments and this will be covered in more depth in chapter 10.

Muscular strength and endurance

The term *muscular strength* is often described simply as *the maximum amount of force a muscle or muscle group can generate.* Muscular strength is normally associated with resistance training programmes that utilise relatively high intensity (heavy weights) and low repetitions (as a result of fatigue due to the heavy weights).

The term *muscular endurance* is often simply described as *the ability of a muscle or muscle group to perform repeated contractions against a resistance over a period of time.* Muscular endurance is normally associated with resistance training programmes that utilise relatively low intensity (light weights) and high repetitions.

The strength and endurance capability of a muscle is mainly affected by the type of muscle fibres within that particular muscle. Essentially, there are two main groups of muscle fibres, *fast-twitch* and *slow-twitch*.

NEED TO KNOW

Groups of muscle fibres

Slow-twitch (type I) fibres (otherwise known as slow oxidative, SO) are the smallest type of fibres and are used for endurance-type activities and posture control. They use carbohydrate and fat as their main fuel source for contraction as they have many mitochondria (structures in cells where energy is produced aerobically). The number and size of mitochondria can be increased by endurance training. They also have many capillaries to supply blood.

Fast-twitch (type II) fibres are powerful and capable of growing in size but are quick to fatigue. They have few mitochondria and poor capillary supply, and therefore use glucose as their main fuel source.

The improvement in performance of each type of muscle fibre group is dependent on the type of training carried out; therefore testing for muscular strength or muscular endurance should mainly depend on the individual's chosen sport or training. For example, it would make sense to test a weight lifter for muscular strength, as the predominant type of training that the lifter would perform would be related to fast-twitch muscle fibres and therefore muscular strength.

In many of the tests described in chapters 6 and 8, resistance is provided by the subject's own body mass (for example in the push-up test and the sit-up test).

Like all components of physical fitness there are many proposed benefits of resistance training. These benefits can vary, however, depending on many factors relating to the type of training that is being carried out. Benefits of resistance training can often include the following:

- Increase in muscle mass, which increases resting metabolic rate
- Increase in bone mass
- Reduced risk of osteoporosis
- Increased glucose tolerance
- Increase in joint integrity
- Improved posture
- Reduction in back pain
- Reduced risk of hypertension
- Reduced risk of diabetes

Power

When discussing or using the term *power* it is often useful to understand the terms *energy* and *work* in the context of fitness or exercise training.

Energy can be simply defined as *the ability to do work* (running or cycling, for example) and the rate at which that work is done is called the power. In scientific terms, power is measured in units known as *Watts (W)*, although there is a great deal of fitness equipment that will show a read-out of the exercise intensity in Watts. The basic equation for power can be written in the following format:

$$Power = Work/Time$$

In terms of resistance or performance training, power can be thought of as the amount of weight that can be lifted or moved over a certain distance (this being the work done) in a certain amount of time. For example, in a bench press a lifter who presses a load faster than another lifter is said to be more powerful.

In order to calculate the amount of work done, the following equation should be used:

$$\text{Work} = \text{Force} \times \text{Distance}$$

Force is simply the weight of the object being moved, multiplied by 9.81 to give the force in Newtons (named after Sir Isaac Newton who discovered that acceleration due to gravity was approximately $9.81\,\text{ms}^{-2}$). If the force is then multiplied by the distance in metres it gives the work done in Newton-metres (Nm). So, the faster the lift or movement of the weight, the more power is generated (as power is the work done divided by the time taken to do the work). In other words, muscular power is a combination of strength and speed.

$$\text{Power} = \text{Force} \times \text{Velocity}$$

It is common for the term *power output* to be used, for example when referring to exercise on a cycle ergometer and, in this case, power output is a combination of the cycling cadence (rpm) and the resistance on the flywheel.

Power is a very important component of fitness in many sports and is often more relevant to performance than maximal strength.

Speed and agility

Even though speed and agility are related, they are classed as separate factors. In fact, research has shown that there is often a poor relationship between the two.

A simple description of speed could be *the ability to achieve high velocity* or *the time taken to go from one point to another*. Speed could also refer to limb speed as well as overall body speed; sports such as martial arts require good limb speeds, whereas sports such as football and rugby require good speed over the ground.

There is currently no agreement, in the sports science arena, on a precise definition of agility (often interchanged with the word 'quickness' for which there is even less consensus of a definition). A classical definition of agility that is often used is *a rapid whole body movement with change of velocity or direction in response to a stimulus*. In a sporting context, agility usually refers to the ability to stop, start and change direction of movement, while maintaining the control of that movement. In other words, agility requires the ability to decelerate, change direction and accelerate again, explosively.

Speed and agility testing within a laboratory or field setting often targets a variety of physical and cognitive components depending on the requirement of the subject being tested. Physical components such as change of direction at speed, speed endurance, maximum speed, acceleration and deceleration are often tested. Cognitive components such as reaction time, movement time, anticipation of opponent's errors or recognising patterns of movement can also be tested. Speed endurance simply refers to the ability to maintain maximal velocity for an extended time period, or the ability to maintain high speed when performing repeated sprints.

An individual's speed, agility and speed endurance are very important in most sports, particularly team sports, but are not thought to have any significant link to overall health.

It can be argued that there are many other physical and cognitive components of speed and agility that can be trained or tested for but, here, only those components listed in table 2.1 will be considered to be relevant.

Table 2.1	Physical and cognitive components of speed and agility	
Physical components	**Cognitive components**
Acceleration	Reaction time
Deceleration	Movement time
Speed endurance	Anticipation
Maximum speed	Recognition
Change of direction	
Limb speed	

Body composition

Body composition relates to the amount of fat tissue and lean tissue within the body; it gives an indication of the subject being overweight or obese.

It is important to measure body composition, not just from an athletic perspective but also from a health perspective, as there are many long-term risk factors associated with obesity. Risk factors can include the following:

- Hypertension (high blood pressure)
- Diabetes (blood sugar control problems)
- Coronary artery disease
- Cancer
- Joint problems
- Respiratory problems
- Hyperlipidemia (high fat levels in the blood)
- Hormone and menstrual dysfunction
- Decreased life expectancy

Even though the number of overweight and obese people varies greatly between countries, in the United Kingdom the statistics for overweight and obesity are of great concern. It has been stated recently that approximately 46 per cent of men and 32 per cent of women are overweight in the United Kingdom. Within these statistics it was also stated that about 17 per cent of men and 21 per cent of women are obese. More alarmingly it has also been stated that a third of children under the age of 11 years will be overweight by 2011. From a health perspective, it is important that the following statement be promoted as much as possible.

'Regular physical activity can reduce the risk of becoming obese by almost 50 per cent compared to people with sedentary lifestyles.' – Department of Health (2005)

Although the potential causes of obesity can include hypothalmic, endocrine and genetic disorders, diet and physical inactivity are usually stated to be the prime causes. It is generally accepted that a combination of an increase in calorie expenditure (exercise) and a decrease in calorie intake (food) is most effective for the long-term treatment of obesity, as opposed to using a single method. Although recommendations vary depending on the source, typical recommendations for weight loss include:

- No less than 1200kcal/day for adults
- Foods should be low in saturated fat, cholesterol and sodium
- Provide a negative energy balance (not more than 1000kcal/day)
- Maximum weight loss of 1kg/week
- 40–60 minute exercise sessions at least five times per week
- Non-weight bearing exercise
- Exercising at 50–70 per cent of VO_2 max

Flexibility

Flexibility has often been described as *the ability to move a joint through its complete range of motion*, and stretching exercises can be thought of as the vehicle in which to help develop that ability.

Flexibility can be thought of as joint specific in that an individual may be flexible in one joint but not in another.

There are many types of stretching exercises. These include *static, dynamic, ballistic* and *PNF* (proprioceptive neuromuscular facilitation), which can be used to maintain or increase joint range of motion.

Although flexibility is a component of fitness that is often tested, it is frequently recommended that stretching can help to prevent injury. There is little evidence to support this notion fully, though, as research has shown that both a high degree of flexibility and a low degree of flexibility can increase musculo-skeletal injury risk.

It is recommended that people with tight muscles would probably benefit most from stretching exercises whereas people who are naturally supple should not engage in more than a light form of stretching exercise.

The most effective stretching occurs when the muscles are warm and therefore an appropriate warm-up is always recommended prior to stretching. A simple description of the common types of stretch mentioned previously can be seen in table 2.2.

Components of fitness in sporting events

The components of fitness and the emphasis placed on each component can differ depending on the sport or event in question. For the purpose of this book we have made the following classifications: team sport, endurance events, sprint events, and strength and power sports (even though it is acknowledged that there are clear crossover areas between the classifications).

Team sport

The physiological demands and fitness requirements of team sport are highly variable. The

Table 2.2	Types of stretch
Type of stretch	**Description of stretch**
Static	When a stretch is performed and held for a period of time at a point of mild tension, it is commonly known as a static stretch. If a partner or another group of muscles assists in the stretching process it is called an *active* stretch. If there is no assistance in the stretch it is called a *passive* stretch.
Dynamic	This relates to stretching in motion where an agonist (prime mover) muscle is contracted to stretch the antagonist (opposite) muscle. Dynamic stretching is usually carried out in a slow and controlled manner in order to minimise the risk of injury and to mimic the types of movement that may be used in the exercises to follow.
Ballistic	Where bouncing movements occur by using momentum or gravity, it is called ballistic stretching. It is usually carried out by athletes familiar with the technique, as there is a greater risk of injury.
PNF	This is a type of partner-assisted stretching so some training is required and it should only be performed by those who are qualified to do so.

duration can range from 60 minutes in hand-ball to several days in test cricket. In some team sport the activity can be practically continuous, such as in soccer, or very intermittent as in base-ball. One example of team sport athletes with contrasting requirements would be a midfielder in soccer and a linebacker in American foot-ball (figure 2.2).

A midfield soccer player will normally cover 10–14km per game, working at an average inten-sity of 80–90 per cent of heart rate max, and perform 20–40 high-intensity sprints per match. This requires many aspects of fitness such as well-developed aerobic endurance, speed and agility, strength when competing for the ball, and power for jumping to head the ball (see table 2.3 on p. 27). As a consequence, testing in soccer players should address these many components and in a sport-specific manner. For example, performing 100-metre sprint tests on soccer players is of limited use as typical sprint distances in soccer are 5–15 metres. Even within

a sport such as soccer there are contrasting fitness requirements between positions, for example the goalkeeper and a midfielder.

Strength, speed and power are very import-ant in team sports involving heavy contact such as American football or rugby union. Over decades, increasing professionalisation has led to large increases in the strength and lean body mass of players, as much training time is focused on maintenance or development of muscle hypertrophy. In these sports, measurements of body composition are frequently performed.

Endurance events

Performance in endurance-type events often relies on sustaining a relatively high velocity for an extended period of time. Because of this, an ability to resist both local and central fatigue is a vital component required for this type of athlete.

The range of sports considered to be endurance based includes sports such as

| Fig. 2.2 | **(a) Typical midfielder** | **(b) Typical linebacker** |

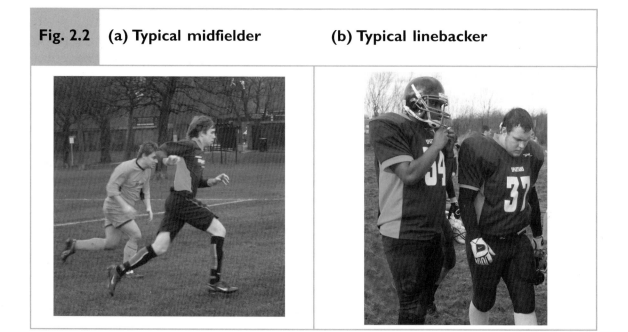

| Fig. 2.3 | **Typical endurance cyclist** |

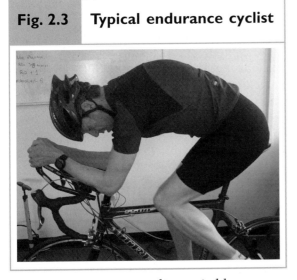

running, swimming, cycling, triathlon, cross-country skiing, rowing, canoeing and kayaking. These types of sport can vary greatly in duration, for example from 10/20 minutes for some events up to an extremely demanding 23 days in the case of the Tour de France. Even though these events are considered to be primarily aerobic (see table 2.3 on p. 27), anaerobic contribution can also be considered important in events of shorter distances or in events in which changes of pace occur frequently, for example as in cycle races.

Testing in endurance events is often primarily focused around tests of aerobic endurance. These are usually tests such as VO_2 max, measures of movement efficiency and indicators of fatigue resistance such as lactate threshold (where each of these is linked to performance outcomes). There is a growing body of evidence to support the case for the effectiveness of strength and plyometric training for endurance events.

Specific muscular endurance (sometimes called local muscle endurance, it is the endurance of muscles responsible for the major contribution to the effort) is also important,

especially in shorter events such as rowing. Despite this, measures of standing jump or vertical jump are often considered less important by coaches and instructors than the aerobic endurance tests mentioned previously. It must also be remembered that not all endurance tests need to be in a laboratory-based environment. For example, in most endurance events, time-trials still have a vital role in gauging true performance levels.

Sprint events

From the many activities which can be classed sprint-type events, here we will focus on 100 to 400-metre distances on the track, up to 1000-metre distances in cycling, a 50-metre distance in freestyle swimming, and sprint kayaking and climbing. Short sprint covered in sports such as rugby and netball are included in team sports earlier in this chapter.

Acceleration and maximal speed are two components that are considered to be of paramount importance to an individual involved in a sprint event. So these two components are often identified as important for testing. For sprint events that last longer than 7–8 seconds, however, there is typically a period of slowing down (known more scientifically as deceleration) so speed endurance and the ability to resist fatigue is considered important for testing in this situation.

Muscular strength (particularly leg strength) is considered to be an important component associated with improvements in acceleration, whereas core strength and stability (and balance) are often considered necessary to maintain correct body position in track sprinting or sprint-kayaking (body position can greatly affect speed).

Agility is not generally thought to be a major factor in many of the conventional sprint events such as track cycling or track sprinting, but it is considered to be important in some

Fig. 2.4	**Typical sprint event**

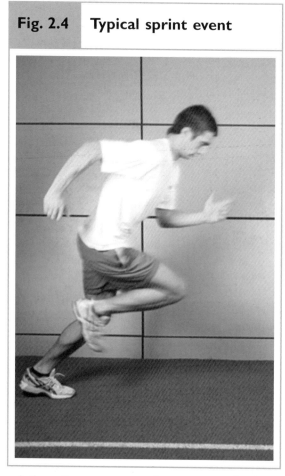

of the other events such as sprint climbing. There are many components relating to sprint events that must first be identified in relation to the event, and then tested for the purpose of establishing either a baseline level or potential improvement.

Strength and power sports

Sports such as Olympic weight-lifting and power-lifting are mainly characterised by the ability to generate great forces very rapidly. Since most of these events involve short high-intensity work lasting only for a few seconds

and have long recovery times, muscular endurance is probably of more importance in training than in competition.

When testing athletes in these sports, some thought must be paid to the typical loads and velocities generated in the sport. How relevant is testing 1RM bench press in a shot-putter when the speeds are dramatically greater and the loads dramatically lower in actual shot-putting?

It may sound surprising but speed and agility are considered to be very important components of fitness in some power sports such as javelin and discus throwing. On the other hand, although not conventional power events, lower-leg power is important in many team sports such as basketball and volleyball (figure 2.5) and is frequently measured through vertical jump testing.

Table 2.3 provides a summary of the main fitness components across a range of sports that you might find useful as a quick reference guide.

Fig. 2.5	**Typical sport with power component**

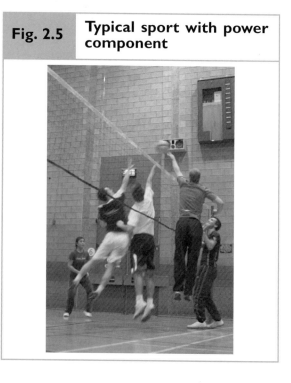

Table 2.3	Sports and the importance of each component of fitness					
Sport	Aerobic endurance	Muscular strength	Muscular endurance	Power	Speed and agility	Flexibility
Sprints	+	++	++++	++++	+++++	++
1500m	++++	+	++++	++	++	+
10,000m	+++++	+	++	+	+	+
Soccer	+++	+++	+++	+++	++++	+++
Boxing	+++	+++	++++	+++	+++	++
Long jump	+	++	+++	+++++	+++++	+++
Tennis	++	++	+++	++	+++	++++
Weightlifting	+	+++++	++	+++++	+	++

The number of crosses allocated to a component indicates the importance in relation to the event.

Energy systems

A basic understanding of the energy systems used during physical activity provides useful information when determining test validity or test order (for more detailed description please refer to *The Advanced Fitness Instructor's Handbook* (Coulson & Archer 2008)).

Introduction

Adenosine triphosphate (ATP) is often referred to as the energy currency of the human cell. The main function of all energy systems is to re-synthesise or recycle ATP.

The term *energy system* is used to describe the source, or pathway, of producing ATP within the body to be used for the release of energy (by breaking the phosphate bonds within the ATP). Essentially there are three main energy systems within the human body that are able to produce ATP (via different, though interlinked, pathways):

1. ATP-PC (phosphagen) system
2. Anaerobic glycolysis (lactic acid) system
3. Aerobic system (utilising fat or carbohydrate as the main fuel)

Measuring the maximal capacity of the aerobic system is typically performed through VO_2 max testing, but testing the maximal capacity of the phosphagen or anaerobic glycolysis systems is far more difficult and controversial. One of the problems is the interdependent nature of the systems. Even an event such as the 100-metre sprint has a contribution from all three energy systems, with the aerobic system providing as much as 10 per cent of the total energy requirements.

ATP-PC (phosphagen) system

The majority of the energy provided to recycle ATP in the phosphagen system relies on the transfer of a phosphate group (Pi) from creatine (Cr) to adenosine diphosphate (ADP) to produce ATP (with a spare Cr) as in figure 2.6.

Fig. 2.6	Re-synthesis of ATP from ADP and PCr

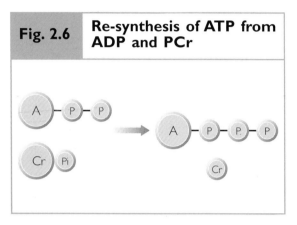

The other main mechanism of providing ATP is the transfer of a phosphate group from ADP to another ADP, termed the myokinase reaction as in figure 2.7.

Fig. 2.7	ADP + ADP gives ATP + AMP

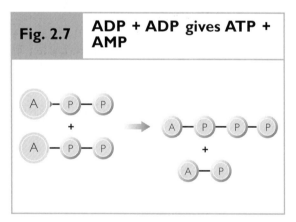

Phosphocreatine is broken down very rapidly during high intensity exercise but is also re-synthesised very rapidly. Four to five minutes of recovery allows nearly full restoration of muscle phosphocreatine stores.

The phosphagen system provides the vast majority of the energy for standard tests such as the vertical jump test, 30-metre sprint,

five-second Wingate and the Margaria stair test, and thus only a short recovery between tests is required.

Anaerobic glycolysis (lactic acid)

Anaerobic glycolysis involves the breakdown of glucose to pyruvate, and then conversion to lactate. It generates two to three ATP molecules depending on whether the source is glucose or glycogen (as in figure 2.8).

Fig. 2.8	Breakdown of glucose

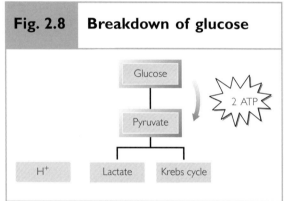

The power output of this system is less than that of the phosphagen system but the size of the energy store is three to four times larger. For maximal exercise lasting between 15 and 80 seconds, anaerobic glycolysis provides the majority of the energy.

Recovery from exercise of this nature takes much longer than that of the phosphagen system. Recovery of glycogen stores typically takes between 24 and 48 hours. So, following a test such as a 400-metre run, it would take a significant recovery time for subsequent tests not to be affected.

Aerobic system

The aerobic energy system utilises fat and carbo-hydrate (in the form of glycogen or glucose) as a fuel, for the purpose of producing ATP to supply the demand for energy.

When energy is supplied by the aerobic system no lactate is produced and acetyl-coenzyme A (produced from the breakdown of pyruvate) is metabolised via a system called the Krebs cycle (also known as the citric acid cycle), and then passes into a system called the electron transport chain in order to produce ATP.

If fat, in the presence of oxygen, is used as the energy source, one of the first stages in the production of energy is known as beta oxidation, which produces acetyl-coenzyme A. This then passes through the Krebs cycle and produces donors, which pass through the electron transport chain to produce ATP (the energy currency of the cell). The by-products of the aerobic system are water and carbon dioxide, which are then released into the atmosphere.

Regardless of the exercise being performed, all three energy systems simultaneously contribute to the production of energy to some extent throughout the duration of the exercise. However, the amount contributed depends upon many factors, such as the exercise inten-

sity. Table 2.4 shows a general overview of the predominant energy systems responsible in an exercise of a typical duration (assuming that the shorter duration exercises are carried out at a high intensity).

All three energy systems contribute simultaneously regardless of the intensity or duration of the exercise. The interaction of the three energy systems changes throughout the duration of a continuous bout of exercise but remember that this will also change if the intensity is varied as with interval-type training. Figure 2.9 shows how all energy systems interact during the initial stages of maximal exercise up to a duration of about two hours (the interaction can also depend on the storage of certain fuels prior to the start of the exercise session as it is possible that glycogen can be fully depleted over a duration of exercise as long as this).

The intensity of exercise is the main determinant of the energy system's percentage contribution to the provision of energy. In other words, the greater the intensity level of the exercise, the greater would be the anaerobic contribution in terms of energy provision, and hence the lower

Table 2.4	Predominant energy systems relating to exercise duration	
Duration (sec)	Classification	Energy system
1–4	Anaerobic	ATP – PC
4–20	Anaerobic	ATP – PC + muscle glycogen
20–45	Anaerobic	Muscle glycogen + ATP – PC
45–120	Anaerobic	Muscle glycogen
120–240	Aerobic, anaerobic	Aerobic and anaerobic breakdown of muscle glycogen
240–600	Aerobic	Muscle glycogen + fatty acids

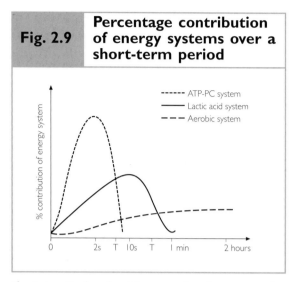

Fig. 2.9 | **Percentage contribution of energy systems over a short-term period**

the intensity levels of the exercise, the greater the contribution from aerobic sources.

When performing aerobic exercise, the lower the intensity, the greater the percentage

contribution from fat breakdown whereas at higher intensities there is a greater contribution from carbohydrate breakdown (this can be important in relation to the objective of the exercise).

Table 2.5 gives an overview of the percentage energy contribution from aerobic sources for a variety of different events. The information seen in table 2.5 is taken from a variety of sources and, as with all research, there is a discrepancy in the published data depending on the source and nature of the research.

When deciding how relevant tests are for a particular sport, it is useful to have some idea of the energy system contribution to that sport. Older textbooks often underestimate the contribution that the aerobic system can make to soccer, netball and similar events. These textbooks tend to quote soccer as being in the region of 50 per cent contribution from aerobic sources and 50 per cent contribution from anaerobic sources,

Table 2.5	Percentage aerobic contribution of a range of sports			
Sport	Duration	Classification	Energy system	% Aerobic
Olympic lifts	0.5–1s	Anaerobic	ATP – PC	~0
100m sprint	10–12s	Anaerobic	ATP – PC + muscle glycogen	10
200m sprint	20–24s	Anaerobic	ATP – PC + muscle glycogen	20
400m sprint	44–50s	Anaerobic, lactic	Muscle glycogen	30
50m freestyle swim	21–23s	Anaerobic	ATP – PC + muscle glycogen	17
800m	100–120s	Aerobic, anaerobic	Aerobic and anaerobic breakdown of muscle glycogen	60
Marathon	124–150 min	Aerobic	Aerobic breakdown of carbohydrate and fat	99
Soccer match	90 min	Aerobic	Muscle glycogen + fatty acids	90

Table 2.6	Percentage aerobic contribution of a range of fitness tests			
Test	Duration	Classification	Energy system	% Aerobic
IRM	0.5–1s	Anaerobic	ATP + PC	~0
5RM	10–12s	Anaerobic	ATP + PC + muscle glycogen	10
Wingate	5s	Anaerobic	ATP + PC + muscle glycogen	8
Wingate	30s	Anaerobic	ATP + PC + muscle glycogen	20

whereas a recent, more accurate, figure derived from video analysis, physiological measurements and player tracking would indicate a value closer to 90 per cent contribution from aerobic sources and 10 per cent contribution from anaerobic sources. However, for the purpose of this book this argument is secondary as it is the focus on testing either the aerobic system or the anaerobic system that is of importance.

Table 2.6 gives an indication of the aerobic system contribution for typical fitness tests.

Further reading

American College of Sports Medicine (2006) *Guidelines to Exercise Testing and Prescription*, 6th edn, Baltimore, Maryland: Lippincott, Williams and Wilkins

Alricsson, M., Harns-Ringdahl, K. & Werner, S. (2001) 'Reliability of sports related functional tests with emphasis on speed and agility in young athletes'. *Scandinavian Journal of Medicine and Science in Sports*, 11: pp. 229-32

Baker, D. (1999a) 'A comparison of running speed and quickness between elite professional and young rugby league players'. *Strength and Conditioning Coach*, 7(3): pp. 3-7

Baker, D. (1999b) 'The relation between running speed and measures of strength and power in professional rugby league players'. *Journal of Strength and Conditioning Research*, 13: pp. 230-5

Berry, J. T. (1999) *Pattern Recognition and Expertise in Australian Football*, University of Ballarat, Ballarat, VIC – Unpublished honours thesis

Borgeaud, P. & Abernethy, B. (1987) 'Skilled perception in volleyball defence'. *Journal of Sport Psychology*, 9: pp. 400-6

Bouchard et al. (1990) *Exercise, Fitness and Health*, Champaign, Illinois: Human Kinetics

Coulson, M. (2007) *Fitness Professionals: The Fitness Instructor's Handbook*, London, UK: A&C Black

Department of Health (2005) *Choosing Activity: A physical activity action plan*, London: HMSO

Docherty, D., Wenger, H. A. & Neary, P. (1988) 'Time-motion analysis related to the physiological demands of rugby'. *Journal of Human Movement Studies*, 14: pp. 269-77

Fulton, K. T. (1992) 'Off-season strength training for basketball'. *National Strength and Conditioning Association Journal*, 14(1): pp. 31-3

Gabbett, T. J. (2002) 'Physiological characteristics of junior and senior rugby league players'. *British Journal of Sports Medicine*, 36: pp. 334-9

Gambetta, V. (1996) 'How to develop sport-specific speed'. *Sports Coach*, 19: pp. 22-4

Graham, J. F. (1998) 'Strength training for elite sprint cyclists'. *Journal of Strength and Conditioning Research*, 20: pp. 53-60

Häkkinen, K., Mero, A. & Kauhanen, H. (1989) 'Specificity of endurance, sprint and strength training on physical performance capacity in young athletes'. *Journal of Sports Medicine and Physical Fitness*, 29: pp. 27-35

Keogh, J., Weber, C. L. & Dalton, C. T. (2003) 'Evaluation of anthropometric, physiological, and skill-related tests for talent identification in female field hockey'. *Canadian Journal of Applied Physiology*, 28: pp. 397-409

Koon, S. (1998) 'Vertical jump ability of elite volleyball players compared to elite athletes in other team sports'. *Journal of Applied Science*, 9: pp. 84-125

Meir, R., Newton, R., Curtis, E., Fardell, M. & Butler, B. (2001) 'Physical fitness qualities of professional rugby league football players: Determination of positional differences'. *Journal of Strength and Conditioning Research*, 15: pp. 450-8

Pyne, D. (Pyke, F. S. ed.) (2001) 'Testing the athlete'. *Better Coaching: Advanced Coach's Manual*, 2nd edn, Belconnen, ACT: Human Kinetics, pp. 77-86

Reilly, T., Williams, A. M., Nevill, A. & Franks, A. (2000) 'A multidisciplinary approach to talent identification in soccer'. *Journal of Sports Sciences*, 18: pp. 695-702

Rigg, P. & Reilly, T. (1987) 'A fitness profile and anthropometric analysis of first and second-class rugby union players'. In Rigg, P. (ed.) *Proceedings of the First World Congress on Science and Football*, London, UK: E & FN Spon, pp. 194-200

Semenick, D. (1990) 'Tests and measurements: The t-test'. *National Strength and Conditioning Association Journal*, 12: pp. 36-7

Webb, P. & Lander, J. (1983) 'An economical fitness testing battery for high school and college rugby teams'. *Sports Coach*, 7: pp. 44-6

HEALTH STATUS TESTING

3

OBJECTIVES

After completing this chapter you should be able to:

1 Understand the meaning of health status testing in relation to pre-fitness testing.

2 Discuss the importance of pre-test health screening and the methods used to do this.

3 Describe the method and the purpose of risk factor stratification.

4 Discuss the importance of informed consent.

5 Discuss the various legal and physiological issues related to children and exercise.

6 Describe the implications that growth during childhood has on various types of testing.

7 Describe the physiological differences between children and adults.

8 List the various guidelines relevant to working with or coaching children.

9 List and describe the variety of health tests (heart rate, blood pressure and lung function).

10 Discuss the issues relating to each health test in relation to the cost, delivery, validity and reliability.

Health status check

One of the most important roles of a coach or instructor is to help subjects to determine their current health status prior to undertaking a programme of exercise or fitness testing. This can help to identify any potential problems that may need professional guidance prior to further fitness-type tests being carried out.

The process of determining the health status of an individual is two-fold and consists of health screening by a process of completing medical-type questionnaires and by undergoing various health tests. Should any problems be identified during either of these processes, advice should be sought from appropriately qualified people before any further fitness testing is carried out.

Pre-test health screening

Prior to any type of health testing (or indeed fitness testing), it is necessary to carry out and record correct screening procedures with all the individuals involved. Although there are many reasons for health screening, according to the American College of Sports Medicine (ACSM) it is carried out for the following objectives:

- Identification and exclusion of individuals with medical contraindications to exercise.
- Identification of individuals at increased risk of disease.
- Identification of persons with clinically significant disease who should undergo a medically supervised programme.
- Identification of individuals with other special needs.

One method of carrying out pre-test health screening is by using pre-exercise questionnaires of which there are numerous examples.

Pre-exercise questionnaire

There are many types of pre-exercise health questionnaires available. The most common used is the Physical Activity Readiness Questionnaire (PAR-Q). Developed by the Canadian Society for Exercise Physiology, the PAR-Q is a short questionnaire that can help to identify possible risk factors for cardiovascular, pulmonary and metabolic disease and is also a useful tool prior to fitness testing.

If any risk factors are identified (by the subject answering 'yes' to one of the questions on the PAR-Q), the form advises the subject to seek advice from a doctor prior to undertaking a programme of exercise or fitness test. If no risk factors are identified (all questions answered 'no'), the form then encourages a programme of *low* to *moderate* exercise to be undertaken relevant to the fitness level of the subject, or sub-maximal testing to be carried out. It is the responsibility of the test supervisor to check that this has been done for all subjects to be tested.

NEED TO KNOW

Moderate exercise has been described by Ainsworth et al (2000) as any activity that expends energy at the rate between 3.5 and 7kcal/min.

Note: The test supervisor must respect the confidentiality of all written material relating to subject information, in particular the PAR-Q form, by ensuring safe storage and private access. All organisations must cater for Data Protection by making sure that procedures are in place to ensure this confidentiality.

Risk factors and stratification

There are many other medical screening questionnaires that can be used prior to carrying out fitness-type testing that are more in-depth than the PAR-Q screening form. These questionnaires can help to identify possible risk factors to coronary artery disease (CAD), which might adversely affect someone undertaking a fitness test if it required a level of exertion. The American College of Sports Medicine (2006) has provided a description of both 'positive' and 'negative' CAD risk factors, which should be identified prior to beginning fitness testing:

Positive factors

- Family history – myocardial infarction (MI) or sudden death before age 55 in father, brother or son. Before age 65 in mother, sister or daughter.
- Smoking – current smoker or quit within previous six months.
- Hypertension – systolic blood pressure of 140mmHg or above, or diastolic of 90mmHg or above, on at least two occasions.
- Dyslipedemia – HDL levels less than $1.03mmol.L^{-1}$ or LDL levels greater than $3.4mmol.L^{-1}$ If neither of these is available, total serum cholesterol of more than $5.2mmol.L^{-1}$.
- Impaired fasting glucose – fasting blood glucose concentration of above $5.6mmol.L^{-1}$ on two separate occasions.
- Obesity – body mass index of $30kg.m^{-2}$ or above, or waist girth greater than 102cm for men and 88cm for women. Waist/hip ratio greater than 0.95 for men and 0.86 for women.
- Sedentary lifestyle – not participating in regular exercise.

Negative factor

- HDL levels – greater than $1.6mmol.L^{-1}$.

Subjects should be asked if they have any of the risk factors described by the ACSM and the total recorded (if subjects have a negative risk factor then this should be subtracted from the number of positive risk factors recorded). The ACSM states that persons who have two or more risk factors, or men 45 years or older and women 55 years or older, have a moderate risk of CAD. It is recommended in these cases that no vigorous exercise testing be carried out unless advised by the subject's doctor. Table 3.1 gives a description of the classifications of total number of risk factors recorded for a subject.

Informed consent

As well as the normal PAR-Q or risk stratification methods, a relevant informed consent form should also be completed prior to any testing taking place.

This form outlines the procedures and possible dangers (if any) associated with the test. There are many examples available on the Internet or you can choose to develop your own consent forms. A typical example of an informed consent form in relation to a battery of commonly undertaken physiological tests can be seen in figure 3.1.

Table 3.1	Classifications of risk factors for CAD
Risk	Description
Low (apparently healthy)	Younger individuals (men less than 45 years and women less than 55 years) who are asymptomatic and have no more than one risk factor.
Moderate (no vigorous exercise unless prescribed)	Older individuals (men 45 years or older and women 55 years or older) or those with two or more risk factors.
High (supervised by qualified person)	Individuals with one or more signs/symptoms of CHD or those with known cardiovascular, pulmonary or metabolic disease.

Fig. 3.1 A typical informed consent form

In order to assess cardiovascular function, body composition and other physical fitness components, the undersigned hereby voluntarily consents to engage in one or more of the following tests (check the appropriate boxes):

- ❑ Graded exercise stress test
- ❑ Underwater weighing
- ❑ Muscular strength tests
- ❑ Flexibility tests

Explanation of the tests

The graded exercise stress test is performed on a bicycle ergometer or motor-driven treadmill. The workload is increased every few minutes until exhaustion or until other symptoms dictate termination of the test. You or we may stop the test at any time because of fatigue or discomfort.

The underwater weighing procedure involves being completely submerged in a tank or tub while breathing through respiratory equipment. This test provides an accurate assessment of your body composition.

For muscular strength testing, you lift weights for a number of repetitions using barbells or exercise machines. These tests assess the strength of the major muscle groups in the body.

For evaluation of flexibility, you perform a number of stretching-type exercises during which we measure the range of motion in your joints.

Risks and discomforts

During the graded exercise stress test, certain changes may occur. These changes include abnormal blood pressure responses, fainting, irregularities in heartbeat and heart attack. Every effort is made to minimise these occurrences. Emergency equipment and trained personnel are available if these situations occur.

You may experience some discomfort during the underwater weighing, especially if you are fearful of being submerged. Breathing through respiratory equipment while underwater should minimise this discomfort. If necessary, alternative procedures (e.g. skinfold techniques) are used to estimate body composition.

There is a slight possibility of muscle strain or spraining a ligament during the muscular strength and flexibility testing. In addition, you may experience muscle soreness 24 to 48 hours after testing. These risks can be minimised by performing warm-up exercises prior to taking the tests. If muscle soreness occurs, appropriate stretching exercises to relieve this soreness will be demonstrated.

Expected benefits from testing

These tests allow us to assess your physical working capacity scientifically and to appraise your physical fitness status clinically. The results are used to prescribe a safe, sound exercise programme for you. Records are kept strictly confidential unless you consent to release this information.

Enquiries

Questions about the procedures used in the physical fitness tests are encouraged. If you need additional information, please ask us to explain further.

Freedom of consent

Your permission to perform these physical fitness tests is strictly voluntary. You are free to deny consent if you so desire.

I have read this form carefully and I fully understand the test procedures. I consent to participate in these tests.

Signature of participant .... Date ....

Testing and children

It is widely agreed that for health purposes all children should engage in some sort of exercise or physical activity. For example, the Health Education Authority has stated that *'All young people should participate in physical activity of at least moderate intensity for an hour a day.'* Further to this, the British Association of Sport and Exercise Sciences (BASES) has stated that *'All young people should be encouraged to participate in safe and effective resistance exercise at least twice a week as part of a balanced exercise and physical education programme.'*

There are many other guidelines that support the promotion of some form of activity for children even though the exact nature may differ. However, the promotion of exercise testing is less abundant due to the potential difficulties. It could be argued to be important nevertheless.

Children and growth

Young children are usually active but the exercise they choose tends to be of an interval nature rather than continuous aerobic activity. In other words, they have short bursts of intense exercise.

The optimal mode and duration of exercise to recommend to children has not been defined, because each child is different in terms of physical and mental maturity, medical status, skill level and prior experience.

Childhood experiences may be important in influencing adult participation in exercise, so you should try to provide positive and enjoyable sessions. Children should also be educated as to the benefits that exercise testing and programming can provide. They should also be told about the effects of maturation on the body; bones grow from the epiphyseal or growth plate (see figure 3.2), which is an area of cartilage near the end of a bone. Bone maturation can be defined as the time when the cartilage ossifies (becomes bone).

Children can continue to grow until their early 20s; however, girls mature physiologically about 2–2.5 years earlier than boys. Growth spurts can occur at different times: in girls typically between 10 and 13 years of age, and in boys around 12 to 14 years of age. This can

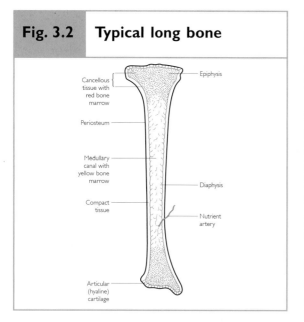

Fig. 3.2 Typical long bone

Cancellous tissue with red bone marrow

Periosteum

Medullary canal with yellow bone marrow

Compact tissue

Epiphysis

Diaphysis

Nutrient artery

Articular (hyaline) cartilage

mean that children are more susceptible to certain injuries as they do not have the bone strength to cope with sustained high impact.

Children are typically at risk of Osgood Schlatter's disease and growth plate injuries. Coaches are therefore recommended to limit the intensity and duration of high-impact activities during exercise or testing.

During childhood, hormone production also increases. Testosterone in males (and some females) stimulates bone growth and muscle hypertrophy but can result in competitiveness and aggression. Oestrogen is also produced which is associated with mood changes and feelings of self-consciousness and can also stimulate bone growth and fat deposits.

Boys' muscle mass peaks at about 50 per cent of bodyweight at 18 to 25 years of age whereas girls' muscle mass peaks at about 40 per cent at 16 to 20 years of age.

In relation to cardiovascular ability, stroke volume (SV) and cardiac output (CO) in children are less than those of adults. Aerobic capacity is normally greater in boys than girls.

VO_2 max peaks around age 17 to 21 in males and decreases with age; VO_2 max has been shown to peak around age 12 to 15 in females, although the decrease after 15 may be due to females reducing physical activity.

Children are not efficient at regulating body temperature, so appropriate care must be taken when exercising or testing in cold or hot environments. Correct clothing should be worn and adequate fluid taken in for hydration purposes both in cold and in hot weather. Table 3.2 summarises the general physiological differences between children and adults.

There are many reasons why fitness testing is beneficial for children and young adults. Just as for adults, testing can help to identify the effects of a specific training intervention so that changes can be made to achieve the best results. Also, some of the tests may indicate potential problems that should be investigated further by appropriately qualified personnel. Tests can act almost as a screening tool to help identify impairments or conditions as early as possible.

Children and legal issues

In order to help increase the protection for children, the government has put in place a regulation that states that anyone wishing to work in a supervisory capacity or in close contact in an exercise or testing environment with children is required to carry out a disclosure check (sometimes referred to in the UK as a CRB check), which is cross-referenced to lists such as the following:

- List 99 from The Department for Education and Skills (DfES)
- Department of Health list
- National Assembly of Wales list

Table 3.2	Physiological differences between children and adults
Physiological factor	Children compared to adults
VO_2 max	Increases from about age six years up to adolescence
Stroke volume	Lower at a given intensity
Cardiac output	Lower at a given intensity
Max heart rate	Higher
Respiratory rate	Higher
Running economy	Lower
Thermal regulation	Less efficient

It is common that the environment in which coaches or instructors work will have in place procedures required to carry out disclosure checks. If you are unfamiliar with this process or require more information relating to this matter, visit www.disclosure.gov.uk. As with all professions there are codes of conduct available to coaches, which give practical information about working with young children. Codes of conduct exist in sport for coaches and in health and fitness for exercise instructors.

NEED TO KNOW

Code of conduct advice:

For sport – Code of Practice for Sports Coaches – available from www.1st4sport.com

For health and fitness – Code of Conduct – available from www.skill-sactive.co.uk

---

Finally, if testing is to be carried out with children then the following guidelines should be followed as closely as possible in order to avoid any unnecessary problems:

- Make sure you have a current disclosure check.
- Always make sure you have parental consent prior to any testing.
- Explain any testing procedures in full to parents or guardians.
- Become fully compliant with the Code of Practice relating to working with children.
- Carry out and evaluate a range of health tests prior to performing fitness tests.
- For safety purposes, perform sub-maximal testing only.
- When analysing test data, use relevant age-related normative data for comparison purposes.
- Always have at least one other adult present when working with children.

Health tests

Even though there is no clear definition of what constitutes a 'health' test, and there are many health-related tests that can be used by the coach or instructor, here we are focusing on heart rate, blood pressure and lung function.

Heart rate

The use of heart rate is an important factor in many types of fitness or health tests; therefore an understanding of the mechanisms of heart rate is essential.

Heart rate is simply the number of times the heart beats every minute (regardless of the environment) and is measured in beats per minute (bpm).

Resting heart rate (RHR) is theoretically an individual's lowest heart rate and is usually taken as early as possible after waking to avoid any external stressors that can affect it – such as illness, smoking, caffeine, prescribed drugs, stress, anxiety and exercise.

In relation to exercise, the response of the 'central command' is to increase heart rate (HR) in anticipation of the exercise to follow. The central command stimulates the adrenal medulla (endocrine gland) to release adrenaline and noradrenaline (stress hormones) in order to increase heart rate. It is common for heart rate to increase to as much as 150bpm in anticipation of a sprinting-type exercise. This anticipatory response is not a particularly accurate system and can often be too great, providing more energy than required. The anticipatory effect can also be observed prior to any form of exercise testing.

Resting heart rate is usually the first of the static tests to be carried out because any other test could affect the outcome. This measurement is useful as it can be used to set certain exercise intensities within an athlete's training. Heart rate measurements could also be used as baseline data for the evaluation of training programmes by monitoring heart rate against exercise intensity at certain time periods.

An electrocardiogram (ECG) measurement is thought to be the most accurate method of measuring heart rate (gold standard) but is impractical and expensive. Nearly all GP surgeries have the capacity to carry out ECG readings using a device similar to that in figure 3.3.

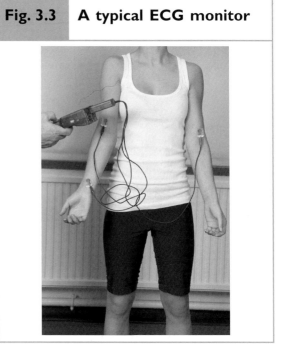

Fig. 3.3   A typical ECG monitor

Essentially, an ECG measures the electrical activity of the heart, recorded at the surface of the body. This electrical activity can be measured from electrodes being attached to the skin (from three to twelve leads are used depending on the equipment available and the measurements required by the tester). Three-lead ECG placements are predominantly used for rate and rhythm monitoring, whereas twelve-lead ECG is typically used for patients in whom cardiac problems are suspected. A typical trace (the printout of the heartbeat from the ECG machine) looks something like figure 3.4, which is known as a *PQRST trace* (this trace is repeated for each heartbeat).

Fig. 3.4 | Normal electrocardiogram

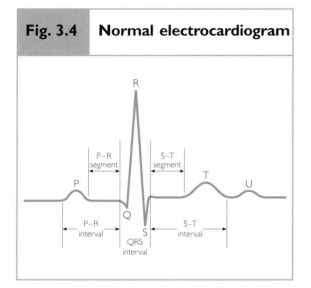

Those qualified to interpret the PQRST trace can retrieve a great deal of information from the intervals or segments. The point 'P' relates to the depolarisation as the atria contract, the 'QRS' section of the trace relates to the depolarisation of the ventricles as they contract, and the point 'T' relates to the repolarisation of the ventricles as they recover from the state of depolarisation. The repolarisation of the atria cannot be identified as it is masked by the 'QRS' section or 'complex' as it is commonly called.

Note: For an explanation of depolarisation and repolarisation please refer to sources such as *Essentials of Exercise Physiology* by McArdle, Katch and Katch.

Typical ECG indicators of heart irregularities include extra beats, elevation or depression of the 'ST' segment (as shown in figure 3.4), or inverted T-waves. These changes can be caused by incorrect lead placement and the patient's medication as well as cardiac abnormalities. ECG interpretation is, therefore, considered to be a skill, which requires considerable technical and clinical experience and is beyond the scope of this book.

Heart rate ranges

True resting heart rate in beats per minute can be extremely difficult to measure so here we shall consider resting heart rate to be the lowest recorded heart rate for that individual.

The normal range of resting heart rate is generally considered to be between 60 and 100bpm. A resting heart rate measurement of greater than 100bpm is normally interpreted as a high resting heart rate and is referred to in medical terms as *tachycardia*. A resting heart rate measured at less than 60bpm is normally interpreted as low resting heart rate and is referred to as *bradycardia*.

Note: These and other diagnoses of cardiac abnormalities must be supported by the use of techniques such as ECG by clinically qualified personnel.

Although the earlier stated figures for tachycardia and bradycardia refer to normal populations, resting heart rates in endurance athletes are frequently below 50bpm and can even go below 30bpm in some rare cases. These low values are mainly due to the large stroke volume (amount of blood pumped out of the ventricle with each beat) that these athletes possess. Resting heart rates of greater than 100bpm may also be due to factors such as dehydration, pre-exercise anxiousness and 'white-coat syndrome' or may even be indications of possible clinical problems. Some researchers propose that a higher than usual resting heart rate can be an indicator of overtraining, but this has not been confirmed or agreed conclusively. A measure of resting heart rate variability has also been proposed as a possible sign of overtraining, but this can differ from athlete to athlete so its effectiveness is questionable.

Exercise intensities set using the heart rate reserve method require an accurate measurement of a subject's resting heart rate. Two of the most common methods are *palpation* and *telemetry*.

> # NEED TO KNOW
>
> The 'white-coat syndrome' refers to the elevated heart rate and blood pressure experienced by many individuals when undergoing physiological testing, particularly in a clinical environment. This can result in misdiagnosis of high blood pressure (hypertension) in these patients.

Palpation

The term *palpation* is used to describe the part of a physical examination in which an object is felt (usually with the hands of a qualified practitioner) to determine its size, shape, firmness or location. Palpation should not be confused with palpitation, which is an awareness of the beating of the heart. Palpation of arteries can be used to measure heart rate but this is difficult to do and can often result in errors.

Required resources

Clock or watch with a second hand.

Fig. 3.5	Palpation of the radial artery

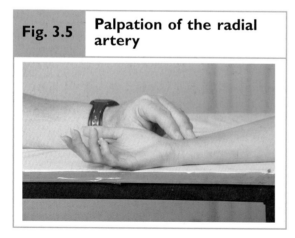

Testing method

1. The subject should be seated and relaxed for at least five minutes before the heart rate measurement is taken. This allows the body to become relaxed and the anticipatory effect of the test to subside, and therefore a reduction in the adrenaline and noradrenaline that would be produced (adrenaline causes heart rate to increase).
2. The tester places the pads of the index and middle finger on the subject's radial artery (just before the wrist joint, in line with the heel of the thumb as shown in figure 3.5).
3. Locate the pulse.
4. Count the number of pulses (heart beats) in 60 seconds.

Alternatively, count the number of pulses for 30 seconds and multiply by two, or for 15 seconds and multiply by four. Palpation can also be performed on the carotid artery in the neck. Care must be taken not to palpate too vigorously as this can stimulate a decrease in the heart rate or even cause the subject to pass out! When measuring pulse by palpation, be aware that the thumb itself has a pulse and may complicate measurements if used. Also this method is often unreliable depending on the skill of the tester.

Telemetry

The resting heart rate of a subject is often determined by the use of a heart rate monitor (chest-strap and watch), which is better known as *telemetry* or heart rate monitoring. Telemetry equipment has undergone extensive research and has been shown to give accurate results compared to the gold standard ECG method of measuring heart rate. There are many manufacturers of telemetric heart rate monitors (HRMs) such as the selection identified in table 3.3. Even though heart rate monitors vary in price, their functions are essentially the same.

One of the problems identified with heart rate monitors is that they sometimes experience interference from other electrical or magnetic sources such as overhead power lines or measurements from adjacent monitors. Many of the more advanced heart rate monitors (chest straps and watches) are coded and hence will only transmit and receive data by the matched pair. Good contact is also required between the skin and electrodes in order to pick up or maintain a signal. As this is sometimes a problem, a small dab of conducting gel, tap water or even sweat can be used to improve the contact and the signal that the chest strap picks up.

People with a small chest, such as children or small-framed females, may find it difficult to achieve good contact and therefore heart rate measurements may periodically disappear. In these cases it is best to use a good, close-fitting chest strap of an appropriate size. More recent chest straps have been made to be more flexible, allowing a better and more comfortable fit so improving the heart rate signal.

In simple terms, heart rate monitors work by measuring the electrical activity of the heart, which is picked up by the two electrodes (positioned on either side of the chest strap) on the back of the strap that makes contact with the skin just below chest level. The R–R interval (the time between each R as indicated in figure 3.4) is then measured and appears on the watch as a heart rate. Variation in R–R has more recently been used as a non-invasive method to assess anaerobic threshold or to diagnose overtraining. Since most coaches or athletes will not have access to ECG equipment, manufacturers of heart rate monitors have developed portable ones that measure R–R interval, such as the Polar Vantage NV (1995) and the Polar 810s. Investigators have found close agreement between heart rates obtained from the Polar 810s and ECG devices (when averaged over five beats the values differed by only ±2 beats/min).

NEED TO KNOW

For analysis of R–R variability, Kingsley (2005) found a good relationship between ECG and Polar 810s at rest and low intensity exercise, but cautioned about the relationship at higher intensities.

Table 3.3	Common manufacturers of telemetric heart rate monitors
Manufacturer	Models
Polar	FS1 (basic), FA20, FT40, FT60, FT80, F7, F11, RS200SD, RS400, RS800G3 (top of range)
Cardiosport	Fusion 10,20,30 – GT 1,2,3,5 – GO 15,25,35
Garmin	Running – Forerunner 50, 101, 201, 301, 205, 305, 405
	Cycling – Edge 205, 305, 605, 705
Timex	Personal range, Digital range and Ironman Triathlon range.
Nike	Triax C3, C5, C8
Oregon Scientific	HR 308, SE 211, 212, 232, 233 (child/female), 300
Hosand	TM GYM system, TM PRO system, TM SWIM system

Team telemetry

In 2001, the Polar Team System was launched to the sport and exercise market. This allows the collection of heart rate data from squads of players or groups of subjects. The collected data can be stored for later download and interpretation. These systems are usually provided in sets of 10 monitors and cost in the region of £1,000 to £2,000.

Although there are many benefits to the Polar Team System there are also several drawbacks. One of the disadvantages is that the tester must, at intervals, check that the heart rate monitor is still picking up the subject's heart rate. Like any heart rate monitoring system, if the chest strap moves or loses contact, the heart rate signal may be lost. However, we have used the Polar Team System many times during training and testing in contact sports such as boxing, judo and rugby union, and still obtained reliable results. Even though this loss of the heart rate signal may be viewed as a potential disadvantage of the Polar system, the coach can view each subject's heart rate in 'real time' and thus if their intensity is dropping or the monitor isn't functioning properly, they can observe this rapidly.

More recently in 2005, Hosand brought out a team heart rate monitoring system (Hosand TM200) that allowed measurement, simple analysis and display of up to 32 subjects in real time. This enables the coach to assess exercise intensity for each team member and potentially provides motivation and intensity targets. This gives immediate feedback to the coach and subject and, with recent developments, can even be used in the swimming pool.

Required resources

Receiver (watch) and transmitter (chest strap).

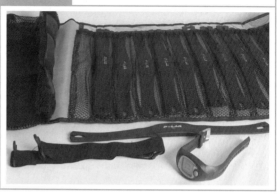

Fig. 3.6 **Heart rate chest strap and watch**

Testing method

1. Attach the heart rate chest strap to the subject (instructions for fitting will come with the strap).
2. Hold the watch near the strap until the heart rate of the subject appears on the watch.
3. The subject should be seated and relaxed for at least five minutes before the heart rate measurement is taken. This is to allow the body to become relaxed and the anticipatory effect due to the test to subside and therefore a reduction in the adrenaline that would be produced (adrenaline causes heart rate to increase).
4. Following a period of about five minutes, the resting heart rate is read from the watch.

Classification

Although, as mentioned previously, heart rate can be affected by many factors, table 3.4 shows a general classification for resting heart rate values based on normal populations, related to gender and age.

Blood pressure

Without blood pressure (BP) there would be no blood flow around the body. BP is primarily

Table 3.4	Normative values for resting heart rate in bpm			
Rating	Women 18–25	Women 26–35	Men 18–25	Men 26–35
Excellent	42–58	39–59	40–56	36–54
Good	59–63	60–63	57–60	55–60
Above average	64–67	64–67	61–65	61–64
Average	68–71	68–71	66–69	65–68
Below average	72–76	72–76	70–73	69–73
Poor	77–83	77–83	74–81	74–80
Very poor	84–104	84–102	82–103	81–102

dependent upon the volume of blood ejected from the heart every minute and the resistance of the blood vessels to blood flow.

The main purpose of measuring blood pressure is to check for any contraindications to exercise. In other words, if a person has high blood pressure (hypertension) or low blood pressure (hypotension) this may prevent them from participating in certain types of exercise.

Essentially there are two types of monitor used to measure BP. The manual monitor is known as a *sphygmomanometer*, which operates on barometric pressure in a mercury element. A stethoscope is required with this machine in order to listen to the heartbeat. The manual method is often referred to as being the gold standard for testing blood pressure. The automatic BP monitor does not require a stethoscope and gives a digital readout of the blood pressure but various automatic machines have been shown not to be as reliable as the manual method.

The pressure of blood in the body is greatest at the aorta as the left ventricle forcefully pumps the blood through it, and varies between 120 and 80mmHg. By the time the blood reaches the capillaries, the pressure is reduced to approximately 20mmHg. In relation to blood pressure there are two phases:

1. *Systolic* pressure, when the heart contracts.
2. *Diastolic* pressure, when the heart relaxes between beats.

The two phases of pressure are measured to evaluate if an individual is within limits. It is recommended that when testing blood pressure, an average of two or more readings should be taken. Similar to heart rate, resting blood pressure is often reduced in athletes, particularly those involved in aerobic activities. Blood pressure also tends to increase with age, so a resting blood pressure of 140/90mmHg would be more unusual in a 20-year-old than a 50-year-old and hence important to be further examined.

Hypertension

High blood pressure, or hypertension, is a major health problem in which the risk of cardiovascular disease, stroke, peripheral vascular disease and kidney failure is raised with increases in blood pressure.

The prevalence of high blood pressure or hypertension is increased with age and is higher in men than in women. More than half of over 65s in the UK and more than 50 million people in the USA have been reported to have high blood pressure. Regular low-intensity aerobic exercise has been shown to reduce both systolic and diastolic blood pressure. Research evidence often indicates that regular endurance training may result in a reduction of up to 10mmHg in both systolic and diastolic readings. Exercise can also prevent the tendency for blood pressure to rise. This preventative measure is important, as there is less risk of heart disease in individuals that have never been hypertensive; therefore it is important to remember the following two main points:

1. Regular activity prevents or delays the development of high BP.
2. It also helps to reduce systolic and diastolic BP by 6–10mmHg.

The risks associated with hypertension, such as cardiovascular events, renal disease and organ damage, can be reduced if the following lifestyle changes are implemented:

- Lose weight if overweight
- Reduce alcohol intake
- Increase physical activity
- Reduce sodium intake to less than 2.3g per day
- Maintain adequate intake of potassium, calcium and magnesium
- Reduce intake of saturated fat
- Stop smoking

Hypotension

This is a term used to indicate blood pressure below normal range. It can be best described as a physiological state, rather than a disease, and is often associated with shock, though not necessarily indicative of it.

Although the effects are not the same as in hypertension, individuals who have lower than normal blood pressure should be advised to move slowly when coming from a floor position to a standing position, as low blood pressure can cause dizziness and in some cases fainting. Extremely low blood pressure requires treatment as it could reduce blood flow to vital organs; therefore it is the responsibility of the coach or instructor to advise a subject with severely low BP to contact their GP.

Blood pressure and exercise

Exercise is often prescribed for people with high blood pressure or as a preventative measure against developing it. The following guidelines should be used when prescribing exercise for people with high blood pressure:

- Aim for endurance exercise training
- Low exercise intensity (40–70% VO_2 max)
- 20–60 minute duration
- 3–7 days/week
- Resistance training with low weight and high repetitions in a circuit format

Although exercise is recommended in most cases there are, however, certain precautions that should be taken.

- Do not exercise if resting systolic pressure is above 200mmHg or diastolic pressure is above 110mmHg.
- Emphasise adequate cool-down due to post-exercise hypotension caused by certain drugs.
- Thermoregulation can be impaired, so be aware of overheating.
- Avoid exercises such as isometric or heavy resistance as this will elevate blood pressure.

Changes in blood pressure during exercise

Blood pressure can change during both resistance training and cardiovascular exercise. It has been demonstrated that blood pressure in some cases can rise to 400/300mmHg during maximum heavy resistance training.

Figure 3.7 shows the systolic and diastolic blood pressure changes during aerobic exercise. It can be seen that arm exercises (small muscle groups) can have a greater effect on blood pressure than larger muscle group exercises. Note also that the diastolic blood pressure is at, or even below, resting levels following large muscle group aerobic exercises. It can also be seen from figure 3.7 that the normal response to dynamic, upright exercise is a continual increase in systolic blood pressure and little change in diastolic blood pressure. An exercise test would be terminated if systolic blood pressure dropped by more than 10mmHg from resting or increased above 250mmHg, or diastolic pressure increased above 115mmHg.

Manual blood pressure measurement

An increase of 20mmHg in systolic or 10mmHg in diastolic blood pressure doubles the risk of cardiovascular disease so it is important that manual blood pressure measurements are performed accurately.

During testing, when the pressure applied to the cuff (as a result of inflation) is above the systolic blood pressure of the subject, the arterial blood flow is stopped as a result of pressure closing the blood vessels. When the pressure is reduced to the systolic pressure and below, blood flows in 'spurts' producing turbulent, eddy currents, which hit the sides of the blood vessels. This results in the 'knocking' sound, termed the first Korotkoff sound. When the pressure in the cuff is deflated below the diastolic pressure of the subject, then the blood flow becomes laminar and hence the noise disappears. The last noise heard is termed the final Korotkoff sound.

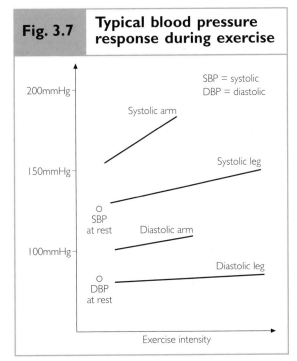

Fig. 3.7 **Typical blood pressure response during exercise**

Required resources

Sphygmomanometer, blood pressure gauge, stethoscope.

Testing method

1. Subjects should be seated for at least five minutes in a chair with their back supported, and their arms bared and supported at heart level. Subjects should refrain from smoking or ingesting caffeine during the 30 minutes preceding the measurement.
2. Wrap the deflated cuff firmly around the upper arm at heart level (the bottom edge of the cuff should be approximately 2.5cm above the elbow crease).
3. Place the cuff over the biceps muscle and fasten, but not too loosely otherwise no sound will be heard.
4. Place the stethoscope over the crease in the elbow (anti-cubital space).

5. Close the valve and inflate the cuff to 180mmHg.

6. Open the valve gently and let the mercury level fall slowly – 2 to 3mmHg.sec^{-1} – noting the point of the first Korotkoff sound.

7. Listen for the first beat and record the level at which this occurred. This represents the systolic blood pressure.

8. Record the level that the last beat was heard. This represents the diastolic blood pressure.

9. Open the valve fully until the mercury level falls to the bottom, as even a small amount of pressure left in the cuff can be quite painful for the subject being tested.

10. If a beat was heard immediately on opening the valve then repeat the test by inflating the cuff to 200mmHg. If this is still the case then increase the inflation by 20mmHg on each attempt.

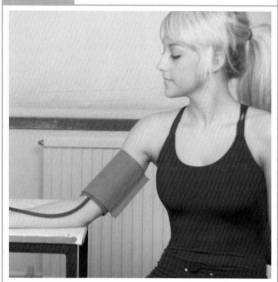

Fig. 3.8 **Blood pressure cuff attachment**

The position of the subject's arm, the fastened inflatable pressure cuff and stethoscope can be seen in figure 3.8, which represents a typical manual blood pressure test.

Even though most blood pressure testing is performed in a seated position, there are occasions where testing takes place in a standing or lying (supine) position.

If standing blood pressure is to be measured, usually one minute is allowed before the measurement is performed. The arm of the subject should be supported during blood pressure measurements, otherwise the subject may be performing an isometric contraction in order to keep the arm in the correct position. This can lead to an increase in blood pressure of up to 10mmHg. In 2003 O'Brien and colleagues stated that the arm position during standing tests must also be at heart level (mid-sternum) as having it above will decrease the BP level measured and below will increase the BP level measured by as much as 10mmHg.

There are many potential sources of error related to determination of blood pressure by manual methods. The tester should be aware of these risks and do as much as possible to control them. Table 3.5 shows a selection of potential sources of error adapted from the American College of Sports Medicine book *Guidelines to Exercise Testing and Prescription.*

Automated blood pressure measurement

Most automated BP monitors use the oscillometric technique, adopting the principles as sphygmomanometry outlined above (except that it measures oscillations rather than noise). This involves automated inflation and deflation of a cuff applied to the upper arm over the brachial artery.

More recently, these principles have been used on the wrist through measurement at the radial artery, or the finger through measurement at the digital artery. In all cases, the limb position is

Table 3.5	Sources of error in blood pressure testing
Source of error	Possible solution
Inaccurate sphygmomanometer	Check calibration regularly
Incorrect cuff width or length	Choose to suit subject
Auditory acuity of tester	Use testers with good hearing ability
Rate of inflation or deflation of the cuff pressure	Not too fast or slow. 2–3 mmHg/s for deflation
Experience of the tester	Gain experience prior to actual testing
Reaction time of the tester	Be able to associate the level of mercury with the Korotkoff sounds
Inaccurate stethoscope placement and pressure	Have experienced tester check
Background noise	Choose suitable environment

vital, as the monitors must be kept at heart level. Correct position is markedly more difficult using wrist or finger monitors and these are not as highly recommended. The protocol supplied by the manufacturer should be adopted, but you should also follow the procedures outlined above for manual BP measurement after a five-minute rest.

NEED TO KNOW

The vast majority of blood pressure monitors available are not independently validated (O'Brien 2001). The accuracy of these devices should not be based on manufacturers' claims but instead on independently validated and published studies (O'Brien et al. 2003).

For top grading by the British Hypertension Society, measurements of blood pressure via automated monitors must be ± 5mmHg in 60 per cent of measurements and ± 15mmHg in 95 per cent of measurements. The British Hypertension Society hosts an up-to-date list of validated devices on its website http://www.bhsoc.org/

Current UK suppliers of validated automated BP monitors include A&D Instruments Ltd, Intermedical (UK) Ltd, Omron HealthCare (UK) Ltd and Tyrell Healthcare Ltd. Prices start at £40 and range up to £150. Boots sell two of the validated Omron models, repackaged as Boots Upper Arm and Boots Upper Arm Intellisense. When purchasing automated BP monitors, cuff sizes must be considered and so purchasing a range of small, medium and large units would be recommended.

Classification

Ranges for normal and different stages of high blood pressure are shown in table 3.6. These figures are related to a normal population.

Lung function

The value of lung function measurements is more obvious from a health than a performance

Table 3.6	Normative values for blood pressure	
	Systolic (mmHg)	Diastolic (mmHg)
Normal	< 120	and < 80
Pre-hypertension	120–139	or 80–89
Hypertension (stage 1)	140–159	or 90–99
Hypertension (stage 2)	≥ 160	≥ 100

perspective. Whether the pulmonary system (lungs and associated vessels) is a limiting factor for performance in athletes is greatly debated. Despite this, diagnosis of obstructive or restrictive diseases in athletes, such as asthma and broncho-constriction, can aid the coach and athlete in developing strategies to minimise the disruption caused. It is useful in establishing clinical diagnoses, assessing the stage of the disease and measuring the effect of therapy such as bronchodilators or corticosteroids (this is restricted to qualified clinicians only).

Pulmonary function tests are recommended for smokers above the age of 45 years or for people with dyspnea (shortness of breath), coughing or wheezing. Pulmonary abnormalities are classified as either obstructive (normal airflow impeded) or restrictive (normal lung volumes or capacities reduced).

Lung function tests are often used as an overall measurement of respiratory function and can help identify potential lung weakness or damage in cases such as asthma. This is a respiratory complication or pulmonary disease (that has a possible genetic link), which manifests as a result of several possible factors:

- Involuntary contraction of the smooth muscle that surrounds the bronchi.
- Swelling of the mucosal cells lining the inside of the bronchi.

- Excessive secretion of the mucosal cells lining the bronchi.

Sufferers of asthma normally experience laboured or difficult breathing as a result of the narrowing of the airways. Although there are many potential causes of asthma, they are generally classified into two categories. If the cause is diagnosed as being a result of exercise, it is known as *exercise-induced asthma (EIA)*. If the cause is related to an allergy of some kind, this is known as *allergenic asthma.*

Exercise-induced asthma

Approximately 80 per cent of all asthmatics suffer from exercise-induced asthma. There are two possible phases of an asthma attack that can occur. These are commonly known as the *early phase* and the *late phase*. The early phase of an asthma attack can usually occur between 5 and 20 minutes after the start of an exercise session. The late phase of an asthma attack can occur as much as 4 to 6 hours following the exercise session. At specific intensities of exercise, cooling of the respiratory tract has been suggested to be responsible for asthma attacks, as has a deficiency of carbon dioxide (hypocapnia) in the blood. Only the smooth muscle contraction is involved in this condition.

Allergenic asthma

Dust, chemicals and antibodies are all potentially responsible for the onset of an asthma attack. During an allergic reaction, chemicals in the body, known as *histamines,* are released from *mast cells.* Histamines are a powerful vasodilator, narrowing the airways by any of the means mentioned previously.

Childhood exposure to allergens such as smoke, pollution and respiratory virus can increase risk. However, asthma developed in the young may abate with maturity.

Exercise is considered to be a key component in the rehabilitation of individuals with respiratory disease such as asthma. Research suggests that benefits of exercise include increased exercise endurance, increased functional status, decreased severity of reaction and improved quality of life. Improvements as a result of exercise can be expected regardless of the severity of the disease.

As exercise can potentially trigger an asthma attack it is important that certain precautions are taken to avoid this:

- Carry an inhaler during all exercise sessions.
- Training with someone is always advisable.
- Breathe in through the nose and out through pursed lips twice as long.
- Include regular upper body resistance training. Exhale on the greatest effort.
- Include regular ventilatory muscle training as part of an exercise programme, 3–5 days per week, 30 per cent of maximal inspiratory pressure, 30 minutes per day or 50 per cent of peak oxygen uptake or maximal limits as tolerated by symptoms.
- The asthmatic should follow a medication plan as advised by the doctor to help prevent or reduce exercise-induced asthma.
- Thorough screening should be carried out to identify causes of asthma.
- Perform an extended warm-up and gradual cool-down in all exercise programmes.
- Running causes more asthma attacks than cycling and walking. Swimming is a form of exercise that results in the least asthmatic events (the air above the water tends to be warmer and contain more moisture), therefore this type of cardiovascular exercise should be promoted above all other types.
- In cold weather a scarf or facemask can be used to trap moisture.

It is possible that a subject may develop an asthma attack as a result of participating in a fitness test (beware as this could occur some time after the test, as in the late phase). Even though the risk cannot be eliminated entirely, it is important that the following steps be taken in the event of an asthma attack occurring either during or after the test (all subjects who have been diagnosed as asthmatic should be made aware of these steps even though they will probably have more extensive knowledge of the condition).

Note: Remember that asthma attacks can be potentially fatal. If the tester is in any doubt they should call for emergency assistance without delay.

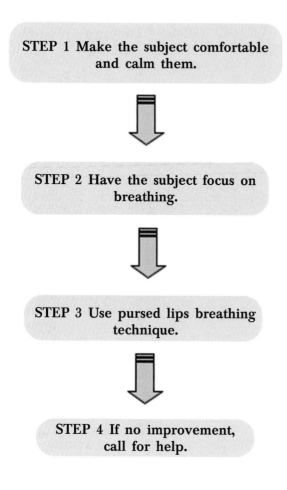

STEP 1 Make the subject comfortable and calm them.

STEP 2 Have the subject focus on breathing.

STEP 3 Use pursed lips breathing technique.

STEP 4 If no improvement, call for help.

Tests of lung function

There are several tests that are commonly used in all environments to measure lung function, or pulmonary function. These tests are known as *spirometry* tests and they measure the rate at which the lung changes volume during forced breathing manoeuvres. Tests include the following:

- TLC – total lung capacity
- FVC – forced vital capacity
- FEV_1 – forced expiratory volume (1 sec)
- FER – forced expiratory ratio
- PEFR – peak expiratory flow rate

- MVV – maximal voluntary ventilation
- EIB – exercise-induced bronchoconstriction

A brief description of the purpose of the individual tests and the units that are used for the measurements can be seen in table 3.7.

Total lung capacity (TLC)

Total lung capacity is defined as the volume of air in the lungs at full inspiration. Measurement of total lung capacity requires a measure of residual volume (RV) for calculation purposes, which is the volume of air remaining in the lungs after a maximal expiration.

Required resources

In order to make a direct measurement of total lung capacity, specialised equipment is required for re-breathing methods involving helium or nitrogen dilution.

Testing method

Since most people do not have access to these facilities, total lung capacity is not a frequently performed test; however, measurement of residual volume is required in assessments such as body composition using underwater weighing (see chapter 4). Therefore there are several proposed prediction equations based on age and height that can be used to estimate total lung capacity.

Analysis

In order to calculate total lung capacity, residual volume is first required. One of the standard equations that are often used to predict residual volume is that proposed by Miller and colleagues in 1998 (note the difference between normal weight and overweight populations).

Table 3.7	Lung function tests		
Measurement	Units	Function
Total lung capacity (TLC)	Litres	This is the total volume of air in the lungs at maximal inspiration.
Forced vital capacity (FVC)	Litres	This is the maximum volume of air exhaled with a maximal forced effort.
Forced expiratory volume (FEV$_1$)	Litres	This is the volume of air forcefully expired in one second.
Forced expiratory ratio (FER)	%	This is the relationship of FVC divided by FEV^1 and expressed as a percentage.
Peak expiratory flow (PEF)	L. min^{-1}	This simply refers to the maximum rate of airflow achieved during expiration.
Maximal minute ventilation (MMV)	L. min^{-1}	This is the maximum volume of air inhaled and exhaled in a predetermined time (also known as Maximal Voluntary Ventilation, or MVV).
Exercise-induced bronchoconstriction (EIB)	% increase or decrease	This is an indication of bronchoconstriction as a result of exercise.

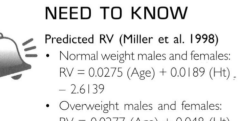

NEED TO KNOW

Predicted RV (Miller et al. 1998)
- Normal weight males and females:
  RV = 0.0275 (Age) + 0.0189 (Ht) − 2.6139
- Overweight males and females:
  RV = 0.0277 (Age) + 0.048 (Ht) − 2.3967,
  where Ht = height in metres and Age = age in years.

Once the residual volume has been estimated by using the prediction equation, total lung capacity (measured in litres) can then be found by using the following equation:

$$TLC = FVC + RV$$

Classification

Normative data reference tables for total lung capacity are not commonly available. However, residual volume, used in the calculation of total lung capacity, typically varies between 0.8 and 1.4 litres for healthy young people.

Forced vital capacity (FVC)

The term forced vital capacity is often defined as 'the maximum volume of air that can be expired after a full inspiration'. FVC is usually measured by using either a spirometer or a vitalograph, instruments specifically designed for this purpose.

Required resources

Spirometer or vitalograph, nose clip.

Testing method (McConnell 2007)

1. Ensure that all equipment is calibrated before use, and free of leaks.
2. Make certain that all equipment is sterilised, for example the mouthpiece.
3. Make sure that the subject is fully rested and fully informed about all the procedures they will undertake.
4. Place the nose clip on the subject.
5. Instruct the subject to take a maximal inhalation and hold their breath momentarily.
6. Get the subject to place the mouthpiece of the spirometer or vitalograph in their mouth while still holding their breath.
7. Instruct the subject to breathe out forcefully, as hard and as fast as they can, until no air is left in the lungs.
8. Remove the mouthpiece and allow 15–30 seconds rest before repeating the procedure.
9. Repeat until you achieve three measurements within 5 per cent (or 100ml) of each other.
10. Remove mouthpiece and nose clip and disinfect them.

Some of the typical errors in FVC or other static lung function measures are caused by incomplete expiration or inspiration, leakage of air around the mouthpiece or coughing.

Analysis

An individual's FVC should be a minimum of 80 per cent of their predicted value, to be

Fig. 3.9	**FVC testing using a spirometer**

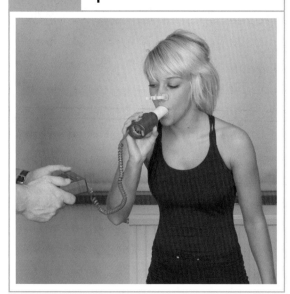

considered normal. Predicted FVC can be determined from the following equation:

Predicted FVC

Males: $FVC = 5.76 (H) - 0.026 (A) - 4.34$
Females: $FVC = 4.43 (H) - 0.026 (A) - 2.89$

where H = height in metres, A = age in years.

In order to calculate the actual FVC as a percentage of the predicted FVC use the following equation:

Actual FVC/Predicted FVC $\times$ 100

An individual's height is a very good predictor of their FVC, and FVC is normally between 3 and 4 litres in healthy females and between 4 and 5 litres in healthy males. It can range between 5 and 7 litres in professional soccer players and be as high as 8 litres in large, tall athletes such as rowers.

Classification

Table 3.8	Age- and gender-related normative values for forced vital capacity				
Age (years)	Male (cc)	Female (cc)	Age (years)	Male (cc)	Female (cc)
4	700	600	21	4320	2800
5	850	800	22	4300	2800
6	1070	980	23	4280	2790
7	1300	1150	24	4250	2780
8	1500	1350	25	4220	2770
9	1700	1550	26	4200	2760
10	1950	1740	27	4180	2740
11	2200	1950	28	4150	2720
12	2540	2150	29	4120	2710
13	2900	2350	30	4100	2700
14	3250	2480	31–35	3990	2640
15	3600	2700	36–40	3800	2520
16	3900	2700	41–45	3600	2390
17	4100	2750	46–50	3410	2250
18	4200	2800	51–55	3240	2160
19	4300	2800	56–60	3100	2060
20	4320	2800	61–65	2970	1960

Forced expiratory volume in 1 second (FEV$_1$)

The term forced expiratory volume in 1 second is often defined as *'the volume of air that can be forcibly exhaled from the lungs in the first second of an FVC measurement.* This test is considered by some to be an indication of the performance of certain muscles used during forced expiration, such as the transversus abdominis, diaphragm and intercostal muscles. The test can also indicate the function of the elasticity in the lung tissue and the possible state of the airways, although direct interpretation is not possible at this stage. As with measurements of FVC, this type of testing requires equipment although it is not too expensive.

Required resources

Spirometer or vitalograph, nose clip.

Testing method

The testing protocol is identical to the procedure for FVC measurement. However, all subjects must be instructed to focus on a hard and fast expiration during each test, while at the same time trying to exhale all air in the first second (make sure that the subject then continues to exhale as much air as possible).

Analysis

The electrical devices used to perform this type of test normally give a direct reading of FEV_1 as a digital readout in litres; however, it is possible to predict FEV_1 without the requirement for any testing of the subject. Predicted FEV_1 can be calculated by using a prediction equation that normally requires only height and age to be acquired. Although there are many prediction equations available, one of the most common for general populations is as follows:

Predicted FEV_1

Male: $FEV_1 = 4.301$ (H) $- 0.029$ (A) $- 2.492$

Female: $FEV_1 = 3.953$ (H) $- 0.025$ (A) $- 2.604$

where H = height in metres, A = age in years.

Depending on the type of electrical device used during testing, it is possible for the results to be given in graph form. A typical graph printout of the result of an FEV_1 test using a digital spirometer can be seen in figure 3.10 in which the volume measured in litres is the difference between 0 and 1 second.

Classification

Once the FEV_1 predicted value has been calculated, the actual measurement of FEV_1 as a result of the test can be compared with the

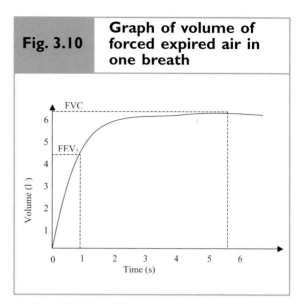

Fig. 3.10 **Graph of volume of forced expired air in one breath**

predicted value. This can give an indication of potential pulmonary impairment or obstruction (see table 3.9).

Forced expiratory ratio (FER also known as FEV₁%)

Once FEV_1 and FVC measurements have been taken it is often useful to express these two measurements as a ratio. This is often done in clinical health environments in which the ratio expression can be used to give an indication of potential restrictive or obstructive pulmonary disease (however, a diagnosis of disease would not be made solely based on this calculation).

No equipment is required for this ratio value as it is simply done as a calculation based on the two previous measurements of forced vital capacity and forced expiratory volume in one second.

As a result of testing, in a normal individual without the presence of any pulmonary disease, measured FEV_1 should represent a substantial proportion of measured FVC.

Table 3.9	Classification of predicted versus measured FEV_1	
FEV_1	Interpretation
> 80% of predicted	normal
66–80% of predicted	mild obstruction
50–65% of predicted	moderate obstruction
< 50% of predicted	severe obstruction

In order to calculate FEV_1 as a percentage of FVC use the following equation:

$$FER = FEV_1/FVC \times 100$$

Classification

Although normative data tables are not readily available for forced expiratory ratio measurements, there are general classification guidelines.

For those individuals under the age of 30 years old, the individual's measured forced expiratory ratio should be at least a minimum of 80 per cent of their predicted value (use predicted FVC and FEV_1 in the above equation) in order to be considered normal. For those over 30 years of age and up until late middle age, 75 per cent of the predicted forced expiratory ratio is considered to be normal.

The value of forced expiratory ratio is thought to reflect the pulmonary expiratory power and the airway's resistance to flow.

From a clinical and health perspective, forced vital capacity and forced expiratory ratio are useful in the early identification of individuals at risk of developing forms of obstructive or restrictive pulmonary disease before symptoms appear. It has been demonstrated that development of severe obstructive lung disease such as asthma or emphysema can reduce forced expiratory ratio to as low as 40 per cent due to a reduction in airway diameter and elastic recoil.

Severe obstructive pulmonary disease can be characterised by a measured forced expiratory volume (1 second) of 30 per cent (or less) of a predicted value, or a measured forced expiratory ratio of less than 70 per cent. Severe restrictive pulmonary disease can be characterised by a measured forced vital capacity of between 34 and 49 per cent of predicted values.

Note: All subjects who are to be tested should be asked if they have been diagnosed with any form of pulmonary disease prior to testing. If this is the case then testing should be postponed until pre-test conditions have been established and implemented. These pre-test conditions can be found in texts such as the American College of Sports Medicine's *Exercise Management for Persons with Chronic Diseases and Disabilities.*

Peak expiratory flow (PEF)

The peak expiratory flow rate can be described as the maximum flow rate during a forced expiration, starting immediately after a deep inspiration. PEF is an important tool for the diagnosis and treatment of asthma and can be estimated using an inexpensive portable peak flow meter. PEF correlates well with FEV_1 and can be measured at home to gauge the severity of the disease and the effectiveness of medication.

PEF is dependent on the effort of the subject and can vary by 20 per cent during the day for an asthmatic patient. A peak flow meter costs approximately £20 and is relatively easy to understand, making it suitable for unsupervised home use, with instructions.

Some of the limitations of the peak flow meter are that the results can be quite variable and it may underestimate airflow limitations in peripheral airways.

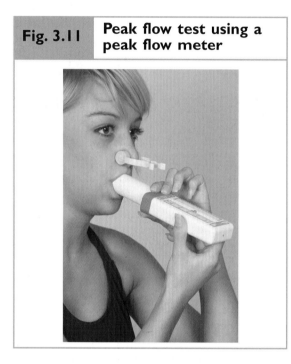

| Fig. 3.11 | **Peak flow test using a peak flow meter** |

Required resources

Peak flow meter, nose clip, disposable mouthpiece.

Testing method

1. Attach a clean mouthpiece to the peak flow meter.
2. Put a nose clip on the subject.
3. Hold the peak flow meter away from the moving indicator, with the indicator set at zero.
4. The subject takes a deep breath in and holds.
5. Place the tube inside the mouth and ensure a closed seal is made.

6. Breathe out as hard as possible in one quick breath.
7. Record the reading from the indicator.
8. Repeat several times and record the maximum score.

Classification

Data regarding peak flow is usually age- and gender-related as in the normative-value tables 3.10a and 3.10b.

There are also several charts available that show average peak flow scores related to height only, such as in figure 3.12.

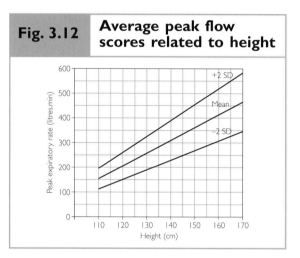

| Fig. 3.12 | **Average peak flow scores related to height** |

Maximal voluntary ventilation (MVV)

The term maximal voluntary ventilation is also commonly known as maximal minute ventilation (MMV). Either of these terms refers to the maximum volume of air inhaled and exhaled in a predetermined time. The resultant measurement is influenced by the strength and endurance of the respiratory muscles (mentioned earlier in this chapter), narrowing of the airways, elastic recoil and distensability of the lungs.

Maximal minute ventilation is usually measured in litres over a 15-second period. This value is then multiplied by four to give a value in litres

Table 3.10a	Normative values for male peak flow rates in litres per minute											
Height (cm)	**Age (years)**											
	15	20	25	30	35	40	45	50	55	60	65	70
191	560	610	645	655	655	650	635	625	610	600	590	580
183	550	600	630	645	645	635	625	610	600	590	580	570
175	540	590	620	635	635	625	615	600	590	575	565	555
167	530	580	610	625	625	615	605	590	575	565	555	545
160	520	570	600	610	615	605	590	575	565	555	545	535

Table 3.10b	Normative values for female peak flow rates in litres per minute											
Height (cm)	**Age (years)**											
	15	20	25	30	35	40	45	50	55	60	65	70
175	480	485	490	495	495	495	490	480	470	460	445	430
167	470	475	480	485	485	480	475	470	460	450	435	415
160	460	465	470	475	475	470	465	460	450	435	420	405
152	450	455	460	465	465	460	455	445	435	425	410	395
145	440	445	450	450	450	450	445	435	425	415	400	385

per minute. Typical post-test values range between 140 and 180 litres per minute ($l.min^{-1}$) in healthy young males and 80 and 120 litres per minute ($l.min^{-1}$) in healthy young females.

It would be logical to think that the more air that can be taken into the body within a predetermined period of time, the greater the possibility of more oxygen being delivered to the working muscles. In other words the greater the maximal ventilation, the more likelihood of a higher aerobic capacity.

This test, although typically performed over a 15-second period, can be performed for longer durations but the inspired gas must contain above-normal carbon dioxide in order to prevent hypocapnia (very low pressure of carbon dioxide in the blood), which can lead to fainting.

The equipment required for this test includes a standard spirometer device or a Douglas bag (see chapter 9) to estimate maximal minute ventilation.

In those individuals who have been diagnosed with obstructive pulmonary disease, maximal minute ventilation measurements are typically only 40 per cent of the age and size predicted values.

As with most lung function tests a prediction equation for maximal voluntary ventilation has been established as a result of extensive research carried out over a period of many years.

Maximal voluntary ventilation can (although somewhat crudely) be estimated by using the following equation:

$$MMV = FEV_1 \times 37$$

Note: This multiplication factor can range from 35 to 40 depending on the author.

Example: An individual with an FEV_1 of 4 litres would have a predicted MMV of $4 \times 37 = 148$ l.min^{-1}.

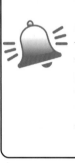

NEED TO KNOW

Research has reported several limitations associated with the maximal voluntary ventilation test. One report has stated that the test is a rather 'blunt object' and does not reflect ventilation when exercising and depends very much on voluntary effort (American Thoracic Society 2003).

Exercise-induced bronchoconstriction (EIB)

It is possible for an individual to have normal pulmonary function in a rested state, but have abnormalities induced during or following exercise.

The exercise to assess exercise-induced bronchoconstriction should preferably be running as this has the greatest chance of provoking a response.

Normally when exercising, reduced vagal tone as well as adrenaline and noradrenaline release induces the relaxation of pulmonary smooth muscle and bronchodilation. In asthmatics, excessive secretion of mucus follows this initial bronchodilation which can lead to airway obstruction and hence bronchoconstriction. An assessment of exercise Induced bronchoconstriction can lead to successful treatment through medication and changing of training practices. This particular test should be of relatively high intensity (75 to 85% of maximal heart rate) and of a duration of at least 6 to 8 minutes. Pre- and post-exercise pulmonary function (FEV_1) should then be compared (post-exercise pulmonary function should be determined over a period of at least 20 to 30 minutes).

Required resources

Spirometer or vitalograph, nose clip, heart rate monitor, cardio machine or running track.

Pre-test conditions

1. Ensure all inhaled air enters via the mouth (use a nose clip) so that it is not subject to warming and humidifying by the nose.
2. Try to conduct the test in a cold, dry environment conducive to triggering exercise-induced bronchoconstriction.
3. Asthmatic subjects should abstain from using medication prior to the test (seek advice for time periods).
4. Subjects should avoid vigorous exercise for at least 12 hours prior to the test.
5. Subjects should avoid food and drink (except water) for about six hours prior to testing.

Testing method

1. Calculate 50 per cent and 75 per cent of the subject's maximum predicted heart rate.
2. Attach a heart rate monitor to the subject.
3. Take FEV_1 reading (as shown previously) three times prior to exercising and record the maximum as a baseline measurement.
4. Exercise for 5 minutes at 50 per cent and then for 8 minutes at 75 per cent of maximum predicted heart rate adjusting the speed of the treadmill or cycle (or other cardiovascular machine) to suit.
5. At the end of the exercise repeat the FEV_1 measurement (0 min).

Table 3.11	Exercise-induced bronchoconstriction classification
Bronchoconstriction classification	Baseline to post-exercise measurement drop in FEV_1
Mild	10–24% fall in FEV_1
Moderate	25–39% fall in FEV_1
Severe	40% or greater fall in FEV_1

6. Repeat FEV_1 measurement at 3 minutes, then 5 minutes and every 5 minutes for 20 to 30 minutes after the exercise (0, 3, 5 10, 15, 20, 25, 30 min etc).

Analysis

Once the baseline FEV_1 measurement of a subject has been taken, each subsequent measurement can be calculated as a percentage of that baseline value. For example, if a subject has a baseline FEV_1 measurement of 4.8 litres and the next measurement value (this would be the zero measurement taken just after the exercise period has finished) is 4.2 litres, then:

$$4.2 \text{ divided by } 4.8 = 0.875$$
Multiply this by 100 to give a percentage
$$= 87.5\%$$

In other words, the second (zero) test result is 87.5 per cent of the baseline result. This would mean that the score has reduced by 12.5 per cent indicating mild bronchoconstriction (see table 3.11). Each subsequent test measurement thereafter would be calculated as a percentage of the baseline measurement in the same way. Once all measurements have been calculated as a percentage of the baseline, the classification table should be used to identify poor performance.

Classification

Table 3.11 shows classifications of bronchoconstriction in relation to percentage fall in FEV_1

from a baseline measurement to post-test measurements. It can be seen that a post-test drop of more than 10 per cent from baseline is usually an indication of a potential bronchoconstriction problem. If this was the case for a particular subject it would then be the responsibility of the tester to recommend that the subject seek further professional advice.

Further reading

Ainsworth, B. E. et al. (2000) 'Compendium of physical activities: an update of activity codes and MET intensities'. *Medicine and Science in Sports and Exercise*, 32: pp. 5498–516

American College of Sports Medicine (2006) *Guidelines to Exercise Testing and Prescription*, 6th edn, Baltimore, Maryland: Lippincott, Williams and Wilkins

American College of Sports Medicine (2002) *Exercise Management for Persons with Chronic Diseases and Disabilities*, Leeds, UK: Human Kinetics

Barnes, P., Drazen, J., Rennard, S. & Thomson, N. (1998) *Basic Mechanisms and Clinical Management*, London, UK: Academic Press

Black, L. F., Offord, K. & Hyatt R. E. (1974) 'Variability in the maximal expiratory flow volume curve in asymptomatic smokers and non-smokers'. *American Review of Respiratory Disease*, 110: pp. 282-92

Boren, H. G., Kory, R. C. & Syner, J. C. (1966) 'The veterans administration-army cooperative study on lung function. The lung volume and its subdivisions in normal man'. *American Journal of Medicine*, 41: pp. 96-114

Bouchard et al. (1990) *Exercise, Fitness and Health*, Champaign, Illinois: Human Kinetics

Brostoff, J. & Gamlin, L. (1999) *The Complete Guide to Asthma*, London, UK: Bloomsbury Publishing

BTS COPD Consortium (2005) *Spirometry in Practice*, 2nd edn, Practical Guide to Using Spirometry in Primary Care

Dickinson, J. W., Whyte, G. P., McConnell, A. K. & Harries, M. G (2005) *Impact of Changes in IOC-MC Asthma Criteria: A British perspective*

Kaminsky, L. A. (2005) *ACSM's Resource Manual for Guidelines for Exercise Testing and Prescription*, Baltimore, Maryland: Lippincott, Williams and Wilkins

Kingsley, M. (2005) 'Comparison of polar 810s and an ambulatory ECG system for RR interval measurement during progressive exercise'. *International Journal of Sports Medicine*, 26: pp. 39–44

Kokkinos, P. F. & Papademetriou, V. (2000) 'Exercise and hypertension'. *Coronary Artery Disease*, 11: pp. 99-102

McConnell, A. M. (2007) 'Lung and respiratory muscle function'. In Winter, E. M., Jones, A. M., Davison, R. C., Bromley, P. & Mercer, T. (eds.) *Sport and Exercise Science Testing Guidelines: The British Association of Sport and Exercise Sciences Guide. Volume I: Sport Testing*, London and New York: Routledge, pp. 63-75

Miller, W. C., Swenson, T. & Wallace, J. P. (1998) 'Derivation of prediction equations for RV in overweight men and women'. *Medicine and Science in Sport and Exercise*, 30: pp. 322-7

NICE Clinical Guideline (2004) *Management of Chronic Obstructive Pulmonary Disease in Adults in Primary and Secondary Care*

O'Brien, E. (2001) 'State of the market in 2002 for blood pressure measuring devices'. *Blood Pressure Monitoring*, 6: pp. 171-6

O'Brien, E., Waeber, B., Parati, G., Staessen, J. & Myers, M. G. (2001) 'Blood pressure measuring devices: Recommendations of the European Society of Hypertension'. *British Medical Journal*, 322: pp. 531-6

O'Brien, E., Asmar, R., Beilin, L., Imai, Y., Mancia, G., Mengden, T., et al, on behalf of the European Society of Hypertension working group on blood pressure monitoring (2003) 'European Society of Hypertension recommendations for conventional, ambulatory and home blood pressure measurement'. *Journal of Hypertension*, 21: pp. 821-48

Price, D. P., Freeman, D. & Foster, J. (2003) *COPD and Asthma*, Oxford, UK: Elsevier Health Sciences

Schermer et al (2003) 'Validity of spirometric testing in a general practice population of patients with chronic obstructive pulmonary disease (COPD)'. *Thorax*, 58: pp. 861-6

Woolf-May, K. (2006) *Exercise Prescription – The Physiological Foundations*. Edinburgh, UK: Churchill Livingstone Elsevier Ltd

BODY COMPOSITION TESTING

4

OBJECTIVES

After completing this chapter you should be able to:

1 Describe what is meant by the term 'body composition'.

2 Explain what is meant by 'direct' and 'indirect' methods of assessing body composition and give examples of each method.

3 Understand the different components of body mass (and explain the difference between mass and weight).

4 Discuss the different compartment models that are used when referring to body composition.

5 Identify anatomical landmarks used in the assessment of body composition.

6 Estimate an individual's body fat percentage based on their body density.

7 Calculate body composition using appropriate equations for a particular subject.

8 Understand the sources of error in and limitations of all techniques of assessing body composition.

9 Identify the most suitable technique for a subject based on time, resources and targets.

Body composition

In simple terms, body composition can be thought of as the amount of fat or muscle within the body. It is generally accepted that body composition can influence both athletic performance and general health, and is particularly significant in sports that have weight categories or when body mass is repeatedly lifted against gravity.

Background to the science

The only *direct* way to measure body composition is by dissection of cadavers (dead bodies). All other methods are based on estimates made from the few cadaver studies that have been carried out and are known as *indirect* methods. These indirect methods include densitometry (for example underwater weighing and air-displacement plethysmography), chemical methods (for example labelled water and potassium counting), body imaging techniques (for example NMR and X-ray), bio-electrical impedance, skinfold and Body Mass Index measurements, and anthropometric measurements. Anthropometry as the technique is known includes measurements such as height, body weight, girth, bone width and body fat percentage. These can be useful, as the size of a person can often be reflective of their health status as well as providing valuable information relating to performance. Proportionality changes that occur within the human body can also have a substantial impact on motor performance and mechanical efficiency as well as on potential power output.

Body composition, from a measurement perspective, can be approached at several different levels where the body is broken down into different assumed compartments.

The simplest and most regularly used compartment model is that in which the body comprises two distinct components, *fat mass* and *fat-free mass* (FFM). This model was proposed by Siri in 1956 and Brozek and colleagues in 1963.

Measurements of density or total body water form the basis of this two-compartment model.

Fat-free mass includes muscle, bone and other non-fat tissues (lean body mass is often used synonymously with fat-free mass, but lean body mass includes essential fats in cell membranes and the nervous system).

One of the limitations of the two-compartment approach is that it assumes that the density of fat is 0.9007g.cm^{-2} (grams per centimetre squared) and is *anhydrous* (has no water in it), and that the density of fat-free mass is 1.1000g.cm^{-2} and has a water content of 73.72 per cent. Fat-free mass density varies greatly depending on an individual's bone density and water content.

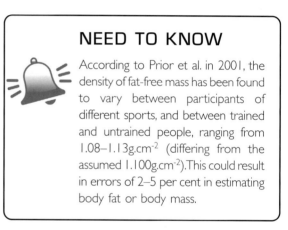

NEED TO KNOW

According to Withers et al. in 1998, these calculations were based on only three male cadavers (aged 25, 35 and 46 years) and most of the error in estimating body composition using the two-compartment approach is associated with these assumptions rather than measurement errors.

There is also a three-compartment model that divides the body into fat, water and fat-free mass (dry), which is a method that controls the water content of the fat-free mass. More recently with the advent of dual-energy X-ray absorptiometry (DXA), a further measure of bone mineral content has been added resulting in a four-compartment model. However, access to equipment to measure total body water or bone mineral content is rather limited due to expense and expertise, and thus mainly restricted to researchers.

Withers and his colleagues examined the effectiveness of the two, three and four-compartment models in estimating body fat percentage in athletes. They found that the three-compartment model improved the accuracy of measurements, but a four-compartment model added no greater benefit than that of the three-compartment model. They also found that the two-compartment, density-based measurements (underwater weighing) underestimated body fat percentage.

NEED TO KNOW

According to Prior et al. in 2001, the density of fat-free mass has been found to vary between participants of different sports, and between trained and untrained people, ranging from $1.08–1.13\text{g.cm}^{-2}$ (differing from the assumed 1.100g.cm^{-2}). This could result in errors of 2–5 per cent in estimating body fat or body mass.

Many of the techniques used to measure body fat percentage, such as bio-impedance or skinfold thickness, are based on density measurements. As a result, even if these techniques could be performed perfectly with no error, they would still be limited by the assumption in the model that the density of fat-free mass is 1.100g.cm^{-2}.

As an example of this potential error, assume an individual has been measured to have a body fat of 13.7 per cent. As precision is doubtful, the measurement should be taken to the nearest whole number, which is 14 per cent (at best). In fact, no measurement techniques (apart from cadaver dissection, ouch!) can measure total body fat much more accurately than to the nearest kilogram.

Another factor to understand is the importance of the *hydration status* (total amount of body water) of the person being measured. If they are dehydrated this will only increase the error in estimating body composition no matter which technique is used. When estimating body fat based on body density, the two equations below are the most frequently used and researched.

$$\% \text{ body fat} = (4.95/\text{body density} - 4.50) \times 100 \text{ (Siri equation)}$$
$$\% \text{ body fat} = (4.57/\text{body density} - 4.142) \times 100 \text{ (Brozek equation)}$$

Height

Height measurement is needed when included in equations or to be compared to normative-data tables. These are commonly used when assessing child or adolescent growth rates.

Comparing the subject's height to graphs of standards of height in terms of percentiles can help gauge whether growth is normal. It can be used as part of talent identification in sports where greater stature is required, for example in volleyball. Differences in height measurement can also produce differences in the relationships between such variables as strength, weight, power output, acceleration and work. This means that individuals of a certain height can be better equipped for different types of activity and team sport positions.

Height varies during the day and is reduced after activities such as running: therefore repeated tests should be at a similar time of day, consistently before or after exercise.

Required resources

It is commonly agreed that the gold standard equipment for measuring height is a stadiometer. Prices range from £60 for a portable plastic stadiometer to £1,000 for a top of the range Harpenden Portable Stadiometer. The height should range from 60 to 210cm and be measured to a precision of 0.1cm.

Testing method

1. The barefoot subject is required to stand erect with heels together and arms hanging naturally by the sides.
2. The heels, buttocks, upper part of the back and, usually, the back of the head should be in contact with the vertical wall to which the stadiometer is attached.
3. The head should be orientated in the Frankfurt Plane as in figure 4.1 (lower border of the eye socket and upper border of the ear opening on the same horizontal line).
4. The subject is also instructed to look straight ahead and to take and hold a full breath.
5. The tester then slides the headpiece of the stadiometer down and into contact with the vertex of the head firmly but without extreme pressure, and the height shown is recorded to the nearest 0.5cm, or 0.1cm if possible.

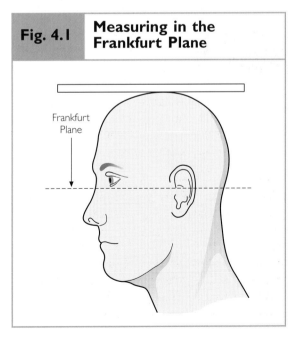

Fig. 4.1 **Measuring in the Frankfurt Plane**

Frankfurt Plane

Body mass

As with height, measurement of weight can be used when referring to normative tables. Remember, however, that girls' bodyweight and adipose tissue levels can fluctuate greatly during adolescence due to changes in hormone production and growth rate. Body mass can fluctuate during the day by 0.5 per cent and measurements should be made at the same time of day, in a similar state of hydration and nourishment.

Weighing before lunch one day and after lunch the next will result in different values due to the ingested foods and fluids. If nude body mass is required, clothing can be weighed separately.

The accuracy and precision required of the scales depends on what the measurements are for. Conventional bathroom scales measure to the nearest 200g; more expensive electronic or manual scales can measure to the nearest 20g. Bathroom scales are not designed for frequent, heavy use and hence are less robust and more likely to be damaged. In all cases, scales must be calibrated and checked regularly for accuracy. Those involved in weight-categorised sports such as boxing soon learn that each set of scales that they use to monitor body mass will give different values, frequently varying by up to 1kg. Scales can be calibrated by using objects of known mass, such as free weights. But be aware that weights used in weight training are usually within a tolerance of 2 per cent, so a 10kg weight might actually weigh 10.2kg.

Required resources

Calibrated weighing scales ranging from £20 for simple bathroom scales to £500 for very accurate, portable scales such as those used in GP surgeries (Weymed BMI200).

Testing method

The subject is required to stand barefoot with minimal clothing, hands by sides, head up, on

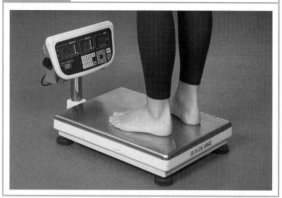

Fig. 4.2 Weight measurement using typical electric scales

a pair of sensitive electric scales until a reading is shown (in either lbs or kg).

Note: If measurements are made after exercise, to estimate sweat losses for instance, it is important that the subject is dry and there is not too much water in their clothes or hair.

Body mass index (BMI)

One of the simplest methods of indirectly assessing body composition in the adult population is by using body mass index measurements.

Even though this method is still used for children, as they develop body mass index becomes a poor index of relative obesity as gains in body mass are largely a result of increases in lean body mass. This is particularly true for boys, but less true for girls aged 11–16 years, where it is a better predictor of gains in body fat.

Using body mass index as an indicator of obesity in the general population is reasonably sound, but in specific groups where being overweight is unlikely to be due to body fat, such as rugby players, it is a poor predictor of body composition. Here body mass index is affected as much by gains in lean body mass as by fat mass.

In all groups body mass index is affected by the size of the individual's frame and density. This method has also been shown to be inaccurate in women who are pregnant or breast-feeding, or people who are classed as being frail. A combination of body mass index and waist circumference is currently becoming more recognised as a good indicator of overall fatness and central fat stores in sedentary populations. Although obesity (as defined by body mass index measurements) in the developed world has increased over the last few decades (1970s–2000s), research in the USA has found that deaths attributed to obesity have decreased over this time. This could be due to reductions in death from heart disease as a result of improved medical treatments and procedures.

NEED TO KNOW

Flegal et al. in 2005 found that the increased mortality rates associated with BMI > 30 were greater in those below the age of 60 than those above the age of 60 or 70, and that losses in height as people age can also lead to greater BMI

Flegal and colleagues also found that there was no increased mortality in those individuals who were classed as being overweight (see table 4.1). This finding indicates that the risks associated with obesity are greatest in the younger population and might also indicate that in the future, body mass index targets should be age specific as opposed to a general classification.

In 5 to 7-year-old children, body mass index has generally been found to be a good predictor of those who were obese, but a poor predictor of those who were overweight. The outcome of research by Mast and colleagues in 2002 recommended that body composition analysis should be used in addition to body mass index measurements for the purpose of screening children at risk of becoming obese.

Obesity has been defined by the American College of Sports Medicine as the percentage of body fat at which an individual's risk of associated disease increases. As a general guide this can be defined as a body mass index of 25, below which the risk is considered low. A body mass index measurement or score of ≥25 to <30 can be classed as overweight and a body mass index of 30 or above can be classed as obese (see table 4.1).

Table 4.1	4.1 BMI classifications
BMI classification	BMI score
Underweight	<18.5
Acceptable	18.6–24.9
Overweight	25–29.9
Obese	30
Class I obese	30–34.9
Class II obese	35–39.9
Class III obese	40 or above

Testing method

No resources are required but measurements of weight and height are necessary. Methods of measuring height and weight were explained earlier (see pages 65–6).

Analysis

The body mass index *score*, as it is normally termed, can be calculated using the following equation for each individual:

$$BMI = \frac{weight\ (kg)}{height^2\ (m^2)}$$

Example: For a subject with a body mass of 80kg and a height of 1.73m, the BMI would be $80/(1.73 \times 1.73) = 80/2.99 = 26.7\text{kg.m}^{-2}$.

Classification

Once the body mass index measurement, or score, of a subject has been determined using the relevant equation, look at table 4.1 to find the body mass index classification. For example, the subject with a body mass index score of 26.7 would be categorised as 'overweight', whereas a subject with a body mass index score of 16.5 would be classed as 'underweight'.

However, be aware that the classification categories used in table 4.1 are published by the American College of Sports Medicine and have been established using data from a normal population as opposed to an athletic population. Keep this in mind if assessing athletes from sports such as rugby or field events as this will affect their BMI score.

Note: Some organisations, such as the National Heart, Lung and Blood Institute, use a range between 18.5 and 24.9 as acceptable/normal body mass index.

Waist circumference, hip circumference and waist-to-hip ratio (WHR)

Both the quantity and location of fat within an individual are linked to disease. In fact, central fat mass (also known as android or 'apple-shaped') is recognised as an independent risk factor for cardiovascular disease.

The use of sophisticated techniques such as Dual X-Ray Absorptiometry scans can indicate the quantity and location of fat within the body. Unfortunately these techniques are expensive and time consuming, and involve exposure to ionizing radiation. This means there is a role for simpler measurements such as BMI to give an indication of overall fatness, and waist-to-hip ratio to give an indication of body fat distribution.

However, WHR is partly dependent on the structure of the pelvis and muscle distribution and has thus been questioned by some as a valid measure of body composition. A condition known as the *metabolic syndrome* is a combination of abdominal obesity, hypertension, dyslipidemia (adverse blood lipid levels) and impaired fasting glucose.

BMI and waist circumference are commonly regarded as better predictors of abdominal body fat and risk factors for metabolic syndrome than WHR. So, while WHR still has some applications, particularly in those over the age of 70, they are quite limited, particularly in pre-obese individuals, indicating that BMI and waist circumference are more sensitive tools than WHR.

Required resources

Tape measure.

Testing method

1. Subject should stand erect, abdomen and buttocks relaxed, arms at side and feet together.
2. Measure the waist at its narrowest point, and then measure the hips at the widest point.
3. Waist circumference is measured midway between the lower rib margin and the iliac crest in the horizontal plane.
4. While the subject is standing, hip circumference is measured at the point yielding the maximum circumference over the buttocks using a tape measure to record to the nearest 0.1cm.
5. Divide the waist measurement by the hip measurement (see figures 4.3a and 4.3b).

| **Fig. 4.3a** | **Waist measurement** |

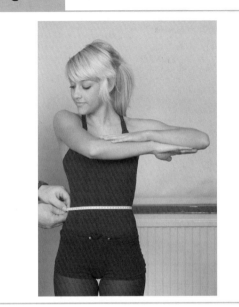

Analysis

Example: For an individual with a waist circumference of 30in (75cm) and a hip circumference of 33in (82.5cm), the WHR is 75/82.5 = 0.90.

One of the advantages of using waist circumference over WHR is that only one measurement is taken and hence this reduces the risk of measurement error. Even though WHR is no longer recommended by the American Heart Association some researchers in London have found WHR to be a good predictor of mortality in those individuals over the age of 75.

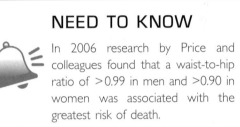

NEED TO KNOW

In 2006 research by Price and colleagues found that a waist-to-hip ratio of >0.99 in men and >0.90 in women was associated with the greatest risk of death.

| **Fig. 4.3b** | **Hip measurement** |

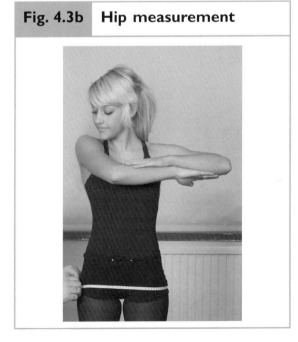

Classification

According to the World Health Organisation (WHO), a waist circumference of greater than 102cm (40 inches) for males and 88cm (35in) for females is an indication of an increased risk of developing type II diabetes, coronary heart disease and/or hypertension. As well as the WHO classifications, there are also sources of age-related risk categories as in table 4.2 that have similar values across the ranges.

Underwater weighing (UW)

Underwater or hydrostatic weighing is the most widely used laboratory procedure for measuring body density. Many of the equations used in more recent techniques to assess body composition, such as skinfold measurements or bio-impedance, are based on measures obtained using underwater

Table 4.2	Risk categories for waist-to-hip ratio scores				
Gender	Age	Low risk	Moderate risk	High risk	Very high risk
Male	20–29	<0.83	0.83–0.88	0.89–0.94	>0.94
	30–39	<0.84	0.84–0.91	0.92–0.96	>0.96
	40–49	<0.88	0.88–0.95	0.96–1.00	>1.00
	50–59	<0.90	0.90–0.96	0.97–1.02	>1.02
	60–69	<0.91	0.91–0.98	0.99–1.03	>1.03
Female	20–29	<0.71	0.71–0.77	0.78–0.82	>0.82
	30–39	<0.72	0.72–0.78	0.79–0.84	>0.84
	40–49	<0.73	0.73–0.79	0.80–0.87	>0.87
	50–59	<0.74	0.74–0.81	0.82–0.88	>0.88
	60–69	<0.76	0.76–0.83	0.84–0.90	>0.90

weighing. An understanding of UW is therefore essential, as you need to be aware of the limitations of using skinfolds or bio-impedance in predicting percentage body fat.

The measurement of density is based on Archimedes' principle that '*a body immersed in a fluid is balanced by a buoyancy force equivalent to the weight of fluid displaced*'. By measuring weight when submerged, a measure of an individual's body density can be found.

UW was used as the gold standard for body fat measurements for the latter part of the 20th century, but DXA scanning is becoming accepted as the new gold standard because it can also assess the contribution of bone.

UW assumes that the density of fat is $0.9g.cm^{-2}$ and that the density of FFM is $1.1g.cm^{-2}$. Since the density of water is $1.0g.cm^{-2}$, fat is less dense than water and tends to make the body more buoyant, whereas muscle and bone are denser than water and hence reduce buoyancy. So, by measuring an individual's density, we get an indication of the proportion of fat mass and FFM.

Air in the lungs (residual volume – RV) and gas in the gastrointestinal (GI) system contribute to the buoyancy so must be considered in the estimations.

UW is a valid measure and frequently performed, but it can be uncomfortable for subjects and does require equipment not commonly available. The subject is submerged in a tank of dimensions $1.2 \times 1.2 \times 1.5$ metres minimum, in a seated or kneeling position. Load cells attached to a platform can be used to assess the subject's submerged body mass. Overweight subjects with relatively large body fat percentage will float and hence a diver's belt of known mass can be used to ensure that they do not float away. Another option is to have the subject sit on a chair linked to accurate overhead scales to assess the effective (submerged) body mass.

Testing method

1. Subjects should maintain their normal diet, avoid eating two hours before testing and avoid foods or fluids that are likely to lead

Fig. 4.4	**Typical underwater weighing**

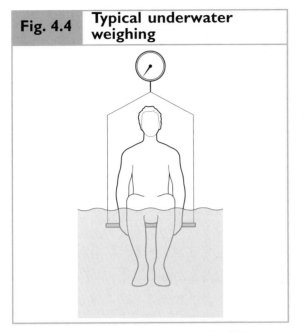

to excessive gas production in the GI system, such as carbonated soft drinks.

2. Subjects should void their bladder and defecate before body mass is measured.
3. Subjects should be clothed in a bathing suit and any trapped air bubbles should be removed from clothing or body hair.
4. The subject should immerse themselves fully in the tank and then exhale slowly and maximally to remove as much air from the lungs as possible.
5. If possible, a measure of RV can be made in the tank following this exhalation, as it will truly reflect the volume of air in the lungs during each weight measurement.

6. This process should be repeated 6 to 10 times for a subject new to the procedure and feedback provided. When the measurements are consistent, no further weighing is required.

Residual volume is typically measured by making a full exhalation and then breathing oxygen in a closed system. This allows a measure of the dilution of nitrogen and the volume of the lungs not involved in gas exchange, and hence the residual volume. If the instrumentation required to measure residual volume is not accessible in the tank, it may be measured in the laboratory. If that equipment is not available, it can be predicted based on height, age and gender as in chapter 3 or by using the following equations proposed by Miller in 1998:

For normal-weight males and females:

Residual volume = 0.0275 (age) + 0.0189 (Ht) − 2.6139

For overweight males and females:

Residual volume = 0.0277 (age) + 0.048 (Ht) − 2.3967

Once residual volume has been measured or estimated, body density can then be determined by using the following equation proposed by Goldman and Buskirk in 1961:

$$Density_{body} = W_{air}/(W_{air} - W_{water}/Density_{water} - (RV + GI\ gas))$$

where $Density_{body}$ = body density (g.cm^{-2}), W_{air} = body weight in air (kg), W_{water} = body weight in water (kg), $Density_{water}$ = water density (g.cm^{-2}), RV = residual volume (ml) and GI gas = 100 cm^2.

Note: Water density depends on water temperature and, at a temperature of 30°C, it is 0.995678

Example: Find the predicted % body fat of the following subject:
Male boxer, body mass 70kg, height 176cm, age 25
Average weight underwater = 4kg

Step 1 Calculate the predicted RV using the Miller equation:

$$RV = 0.0275 \text{ (Age)} + 0.0189 \text{ (Ht)} - 2.6139$$
$$= 1.40 \text{ litres}$$
$$\text{Therefore } RV = 1.40 \text{ litres}$$

Step 2 The next step is to calculate body density using the equation proposed by Goldman and Buskirk:

$$\text{body density} = W_{air}/(W_{air} - W_{water}/\text{Density}_{water} - (RV + GI \text{ gas})$$
$$= 70/(70 - 4/0.995678 - (1.4 + 0.1))$$
$$= 70/(66.29 - 1.5)$$
$$= 1.080 \text{g/cm}^2$$
$$\text{Therefore body density} = 1.080 \text{g/cm}^2$$

Step 3 Estimate % body fat based on body density using the two equations below, which are the most frequently used and researched.

% body fat = $(4.95/\text{body density} - 4.50) \times 100$ (Siri equation)

% body fat = $(4.57/\text{body density} - 4.142) \times 100$ (Brozek equation)

So predicted % body fat using the Siri equation is:

$$\text{% body fat} = (4.95/1.080 - 4.50) \times 100$$
$$= (4.58 - 4.5) \times 100$$
$$= 8.1$$
$$\text{Therefore body fat} = 8.1\%$$

Predicted % body fat using the Brozek equation is:

$$\text{% body fat} = (4.57/1.080 - 4.142) \times 100$$
$$= (4.239 - 4.142) \times 100$$
$$= 9.7$$
$$\text{Therefore body fat} = 9.7\%$$

There are many potential errors in this calculation of percentage body fat. As outlined in the previous example, there is an assumption of standard densities for fat and fat-free mass, which in fact, as explained earlier, can vary from individual to individual. As a predictor of body fat percentage, the example calculation can be improved by calculating the measurement of total body water (see below). The other errors associated with this particular example are in the accurate determination of submerged weight and the measurement of residual volume. An error of 0.05kg in estimating submerged weight will increase or decrease the outcome of body fat percentage by 0.5 per cent, whereas an error of 0.2 litres in estimating residual volume will increase or decrease body fat percentage by 1 per cent. There are many possible errors associated with this type of measurement that could be compounded to give an inaccurate outcome.

Total body water (TBW) estimation

Since fat mass is relatively low in water and fat-free mass is high in water, an estimation of total body water (TBW) can be used to calculate fat-free mass and hence percentage body fat. This would help reduce errors associated with body fat percentage measurements.

One method in which body water can be measured is by the dilution of tracers such as deuterium oxide (D_2O).

> ### NEED TO KNOW
> Research by Lukaski and Johnson in 1985 has shown that deuterium oxide can be used extensively because its distribution follows that of water and it is non-toxic in small amounts and non-radioactive.

By measuring how much the deuterium oxide is diluted in the body, it is possible to estimate the total body water. This is typically obtained by the subject ingesting 10g of deuterium oxide in 300ml of water, waiting three hours for the tracer to equilibrate and then taking a urine or saliva sample from that subject. The deuterium oxide concentration in the urine passed by the subject is then analysed by a technique called mass spectroscopy.

Since fat-free mass is estimated to be 73.2 per cent water, fat-free mass can be estimated and from this an estimation of percentage body fat.

The errors in estimating total body water lead to an uncertainty of typically 2–3 per cent in body fat measurements.

This type of analysis can be costly and time-consuming, requiring specific equipment, and is only really practical for scientific research. The modified equation proposed by Siri in 1961 for estimating percentage body fat is as follows:

$$\% \text{ body fat} = [(2.1176/\text{body density}) - (0.78 \times \text{TBW}) - 1.351] \times 100$$

Advanced techniques

These advanced techniques require the use of relatively sophisticated devices, complex calculations or a high degree of competency by the tester. Techniques include DXA scanning, air displacement, bio-electrical impedance, infra-red reactance, anthropometry and skinfolds.

DXA scanning

Dual-energy x-ray absorptiometry (DXA) was originally designed to measure bone density. It works by analysing the passing of x-rays with low energy and high energy through the body. The passing of these x-rays depends on the composition of the tissues. More frequently, new devices used to assess body composition are validated using DXA scans as the gold standard or criterion method.

DXA measurements commonly take only 5–10 minutes, are non-invasive, precise and independent of the operator. They can also be used to assess the location of body fat and fat-free mass. Scanning includes very accurate measures of bone mineral content and is more precise for fat-free mass than other techniques (measurement error of 1kg). In terms of body fat percentage, the error is approximately 3 per cent. The cost of measurement is minimal but the main disadvantage is the cost of the equipment as a DXA scanner costs approximately £50,000. Another disadvantage is that, for obese individuals, some scanners are not large enough, and hence they cannot be fully scanned in one go. This type of equipment is mainly restricted to clinical environments or university laboratories and therefore not easily accessible to the general public.

Air-displacement plethysmography (BODPOD)

Air-displacement plethysmography works on the relationship between gas and volume, from which pressure measurements can be used to estimate the volume of the subject. The subject's body mass is then accurately measured and density can then be calculated as mass/volume. Body fat percentage can then be estimated according to the equations of Siri or Brozek described previously.

The gas volume in the thorax is estimated during this procedure to include it in the assessment of body volume.

One of the leading product names related to this type of testing is BODPOD, which is often the term used to describe air-displacement plethysmography. Body density assessed using BODPOD tends to be greater than that obtained from underwater weighing and hence slightly lower body fat percentages are obtained.

| Fig. 4.5 | **Typical BODPOD** |

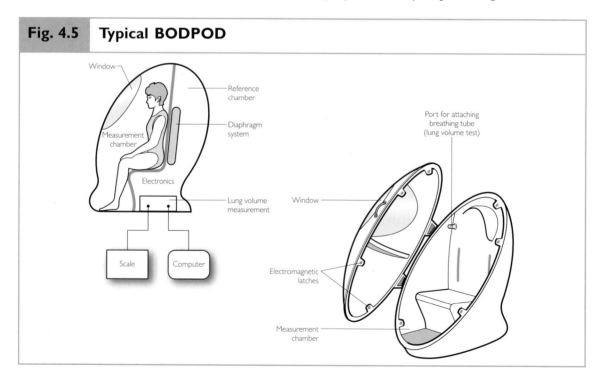

In contrast, it tends to provide higher percentage fat values than DXA scans.

Some advantages are the ease and comfort of use for subjects. Disadvantages are equipment costs and that it is sensitive to temperature and pressure changes in the room where the measurements are made.

Electrical impedance (bio-impedance)

The previous description of total body water was provided because it forms the basis in estimating body fat using bio-impedance analysis, and it helps to highlight some of the limitations of the bio-impedance technique.

Bio-electrical impedance analysis is becoming a more frequently used method to assess body composition due to its ease of use, portability and cost. It is based on the principle that the resistance to a current is inversely related to the fat-free mass contained within the body. In other words, the greater the fat-free mass in the body, the lower the resistance.

The fat-free mass contains virtually all the water and electrolytes in the body and hence conducts most of the electric current produced by the bioelectrical device. Fat mass, on the other hand, is very low in water and electrolytes, and resists the flow of electric current.

This small current (usually 0.4–0.8 amps) is passed between surface electrodes on a hand and foot, and measures the impedance to this current at either single (usually 50kHz) or multiple (5kHz–1Mhz) frequencies.

The standard error of measurement is 2–4kg for fat-free mass and the analysers are relatively easy to use. Commercially available analysers range from £30 to several thousand pounds. Many portable handheld analysers are not independently validated.

As outlined previously, the measurement of resistance is quite simple as the analyser contains a series of processors that convert a measure of resistance to total body water, fat-free mass and then to body fat percentage. Better analysers will provide the equations used to calculate body fat percentage and an option for selecting for different populations, such as the obese. These equations are very often not provided as they are referred to as 'trade secrets' and not revealed. Another vital value is a measure of the impedance (related to resistance) in ohms, which can then be used with prediction equations.

One of the limitations with bio-impedance is that prediction equations developed with one analyser may not be valid using impedance values obtained from another analyser.

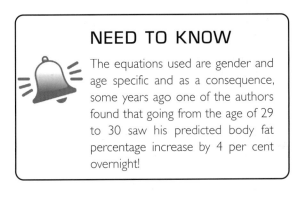

NEED TO KNOW

The equations used are gender and age specific and as a consequence, some years ago one of the authors found that going from the age of 29 to 30 saw his predicted body fat percentage increase by 4 per cent overnight!

Bio-impedance values are largely determined by the body water of the subject being tested and hence this must be standardised before any testing takes place.

Testing should be performed before exercise and not dehydrated because impedance is affected by fluid loss, changes in body temperature and sweat on the hands and legs.

Electrodes are positioned relative to anatomical landmarks on the foot/ankle and hand/wrist. This positioning is vital as changes can dramatically affect the body fat measurements provided.

Bio-impedance measurements of body fat are highly reproducible and very similar measurements are obtained by different analysers providing the protocol is followed correctly.

The training involved is very simple and can be followed from the manual, which makes it an appealing option for many coaches or instructors. Despite this, care must be taken and the accuracy of the measurements obtained is sometimes questionable.

Testing methods (standard bio-impedance)

There are several impedance analysers available on the market. The procedure for measurement is fairly simple but regardless of the analyser used, the following preparation before testing, as recommended by Heyward in 1996, should be followed.

- No eating or drinking in the four hours before the test
- No exercise for 12 hours before the test
- Urinate within 30 minutes before the test
- No alcohol consumption within 48 hours of the test
- No diuretics within seven days before the test

Test

1. Ensure that the analyser is calibrated before using. This is usually done by comparing the resistance obtained by the analyser to a calibration resistor of known resistance (usually 500Ω).
2. Subject should lie on a non-conductive surface (if you use a metal bench, ensure that it is covered with blankets and sheets).
3. Legs should be positioned so that the thighs do not touch, and hands should not touch the torso.
4. Position the electrodes with reference to the manufacturer's recommendations. This is usually relative to anatomical landmarks such as the ulnar head (figure 4.6a) and medial malleolus (figure 4.6b) (middle finger and middle toe).
5. The electrode sites should be cleaned to reduce loss of signal and, depending on the

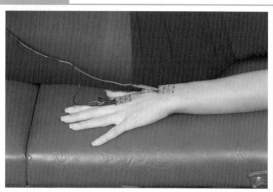

Fig. 4.6a Electrode hand connections

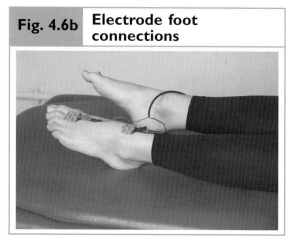

Fig. 4.6b Electrode foot connections

type of electrode used, a conducting gel should be placed between the electrodes and the skin.
6. The source electrode produces the current and the reference (detecting) electrode detects it. The drop in voltage between the two reference electrodes determines the impedance.

Near infra-red reactance (NIR)

The method known as near infra-red reactance (NIR) involves the emission of an infra-red light (a term for a specific wavelength region of the spectrum of light) into specific sites on the body (normally the bicep muscle in the arm). The amount of light absorbed and reflected by the body is assumed to be related to the composition of the body tissue and the infra-red wavelengths used.

Peak absorption of infra-red light has been found to occur at 930 nanometres (a nanometre $= 10^{-9}$ metres) for pure fat and at 970 nanometres for pure water. Usually five to six wavelengths (near infra-red) are used in infra-red devices and body fat percentage is then estimated from height and weight (entered into the device), and the optical density values recorded.

Similar to bio-electrical impedance devices, manufacturers rarely provide the equations used in the calculation of percentage body fat; however, the technical error associated with the measurements when using near infra-red reactance devices is typically in the region of 4 per cent.

NEED TO KNOW

Investigators have found that near infra-red reactance and bio-electrical impedance are reliable and valid for the estimation of body mass and slightly better than measures of height and body mass alone (Fornetti et al. 1999).

One of the leading manufacturers of near infra-red reactance devices is a company called Futrex whose products ranges from approximately £100 for the Futrex 1100 to £3,000 for the Futrex 6100. The Futrex 6100 device uses different frequencies than the Futrex 1100 and has been found to reduce the error in associated measurement.

One of the advantages of using a near infra-red reactance device to estimate body composition is that it is lightweight and portable. Another

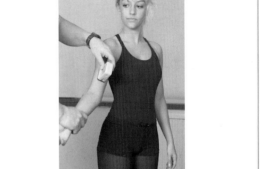

Fig. 4.7 Using a typical infra-red reactance device

commonly agreed advantage is that it is easy to use and non-invasive. Research, on the other hand, has demonstrated that there will always be a limitation to using a single-site method (biceps) to estimate overall body fat.

Like many other methods of assessing body composition, it is also highly likely that the predictions of body fat are as much related to the subject's height, weight and gender inputted into the device as to the absorption measures recorded. Again, this is difficult to assess without the equations provided, as these are not supplied by the manufacturer. Unlike skinfold measurement, for instance, it is not possible to use newly improved equations for estimating body fat percentage or equations that are more relevant for the subjects being tested. For example, to assess body fat percentage in obese females over the age of 60, it would be an advantage if the population used to derive the prediction equations was similar, or at least included, when the equations were developed.

Testing method

There are several reactance devices available on the market. The following outlines the protocol for a typical single-site device, which gives a reading of body fat percentage.

1. Press the 'on' button.
2. Enter the subject's height in centimetres by pressing the 'weight/height' key to increase the value, and pressing the 'weight/height' key in conjunction with the 'function/measure' key to decrease the value. Press 'enter' when the correct value is obtained.
3. Enter the subject's weight in kilograms using the same approach as above, and then press the 'enter' key. The display should read 'std'. With the optical standard cap still attached to the device press the 'enter' key. The display will change to '1' when calibration is complete. The cap can now be removed.
4. Place the device perpendicular across the midpoint of the biceps brachii muscles with the display facing the shoulder. The device should be pressed down so the sensor window is touching the skin and the biceps muscle should be relaxed.
5. With the device in place against the arm, press the 'function/measure' button once. The display will change to '2'.
6. Remove the device from the arm then reposition in the same place on the arm.
7. Press 'function/measure' again.
8. A value for percentage body fat will then be displayed.

Note: Press 'enter' to set the variables for the next subject and repeat the procedure

Anthropometry

The term *anthropometry* simply refers to the science relating to the measurement of body mass and proportions of the human body (see table 4.3 for more details). This type of measurement can also produce estimated measures of bone, muscle and adipose tissue.

There are many potential errors in the estimation of body composition associated with anthropometric measurement methods. One of these is that the techniques used are often based on other indirect measures of body composition, which have their own inherent errors. In previous decades, the indirect measurement of popular choice was underwater weighing, but nowadays measurements using DXA-based equations are becoming more popular.

Another area of concern is the skill involved in accurate identification of the points from which to measure girths or skinfolds, especially in the obese population. These measurement points are more accurately known as landmarks and refer to skeletal points that lie close to the body surface. These landmarks are used to locate the measurement sites (landmarks are found through palpation with the thumb and fingers of the left hand, allowing the right hand to make the marks with a felt-tip pen) relevant to the particular method used.

There is a lack of standardised, accepted measures with this technique. It can often be seen in research that different investigators label the same sites in different ways. Within the UK and many other countries there is growing acceptance of the International Society for the Advancement of Kinanthropometry (ISAK), which has accurately identified the methods of locating the most commonly used skinfold and girth sites.

Table 4.3	Information provided by anthropometric techniques
Technique	Information provided
Skinfolds (mm)	Adipose tissue and hence FFM
Circumferences (girths) (cm)	Muscle mass, limb volumes, skeletal size and adipose tissue
Diameters (cm)	Mainly skeletal size

Two major advantages of anthropometry are the relatively low expense (usually only a tape measure is required) and the versatility offered compared to other techniques.

Body-part girth and diameter measurements can also be a useful tool for coaches and instructors in the estimation of body composition and changes in segment and trunk volumes. The value and importance (based on specific research) of measurements such as waist and hip circumference is mentioned in earlier sections.

Skinfolds

It is generally considered that in the adult population, 50–70 per cent of adipose tissue is located subcutaneously (under the skin). The subcutaneous fat deposit is assumed to be related to the deeper fat stores of the body and, because

of this, the vast majority of approaches to assessing body composition are made using skinfold measurements with a device known as a skinfold calliper. This is simply a device used to grip fat tissue at various sites on the body.

The location of the skinfold site (point at which a skinfold measurement is taken) is vital, as differences of as little as a centimetre can affect the values obtained for subjects, especially for sites around the abdominal area.

There are several types of skinfold calliper available. It is important which one you choose, as the calliper type can affect the readings obtained.

The calliper must be calibrated to a constant pressure (usually $10g.mm^{-2}$) and have a scale that can be read to 1mm where possible. Harpenden, Lange and Holtain are three of the most accepted brands of calliper and cost £100–200 to purchase. Cheaper plastic callipers such as the Slimguide

Table 4.4	Skinfold sites of various methods				
Skinfold sites	Jackson et al. (1980) ∑3, female	Jackson & Pollock (1978) ∑3, male	Jackson et al. (1980) ∑7, female	Jackson & Pollock (1978) ∑7, male	Durnin & Womersley (1974) ∑4, male
Pectoral		X	X	X	
Midaxillary			X	X	
Abdominal		X	X	X	
Iliac crest					X
Suprailium	X		X	X	
Subscapular			X	X	X
Triceps	X		X	X	X
Biceps					X
Mid-thigh	X	X	X	X	

Modified from Hawes and Martin (2001)

Note: The term ∑ refers to the sum of, for example ∑3 and ∑7 refer to the sum of 3 and 7 sites respectively.

are widely used and, while less accurate and robust than Harpenden callipers, they are useful for training and cost approximately £15.

One of the limitations of skinfold measurement is that while the distribution of fat around the body can be categorised as *android* (mainly around the centre) and *gynoid* (hips and thighs), it is in fact highly variable between individuals.

The basis of traditional equations for determining body fat percentage using the skinfold method is to convert a series of skinfold measurements, taken from various sites on the body, into a measure of that individual's body density.

There are many methods of skinfold assessment that have been validated over the years. Table 4.4 gives a selection of methods used and the relevant sites assessed for that method.

Depending on the skinfold method used, the value for body density is taken to estimate the percentage of body fat using either the Siri or Brozek equation (specific equations developed for estimating body fat percentage from body density).

When choosing an equation to estimate body fat percentage using skinfolds, select one that has been developed using a similar population to the subject in terms of age, gender, athletic status, ethnicity etc.

Men with the same sum of skinfolds as a female tend to have a greater body density due to the higher bone density and greater muscle mass in males and thus the equations are gender specific.

If possible, it may be more useful to choose an equation that has skinfolds from a variety of sites such as the arm, leg, and trunk. Raw scores are frequently used when measuring skinfolds, but most subjects will be interested in getting a predicted body fat percentage based on the skinfold measurement, however big the potential for error in those predictions.

There are over 100 equations available for the estimation of body composition, which may seem overwhelming to those new to anthropometry. For the purposes of this book, we are selecting several equations, which are commonly used and

Table 4.5	Equations for sample skinfold methods	
Protocol	Equation	Group
Durnin and Womersley (1974)	body density = $1.1610 - 0.0632\log\sum 4$ sites body density = $1.1581 - 0.0720\log\sum 4$ sites body density = $1.1533 - 0.0643\log\sum 4$ sites body density = $1.1369 - 0.0598\log\sum 4$ sites	Men Women Boys Girls
Jackson & Pollock (1978) three sites	body density = $1.1093800 - 0.0008267(\sum 3)$ $+ 0.0000016(\sum 3)2 - 0.0002574$(age in years)	Males
Jackson et al. (1980) – three sites	body density = $1.1099421 - 0.0009929(\sum 3)$ $+ 0.0000016(\sum 3)2 - 0.0001392$(age in years)	Females
Jackson & Pollock (1978) – seven sites	body density = $1.112 - 0.00043499(\sum 7) +$ $0.00000055(\sum 7)2 - 0.00028826$(age in years)	Males
Jackson et al. (1980) – seven sites	body density = $1.1097 - 0.00046971(\sum 7) +$ $0.00000056(\sum 7)2 - 0.00012828$(age in years)	Females

Note: $\sum 3$, $\sum 4$ and $\sum 7$ means the sum of the three, four or seven skin-folds (sites) to be used for each prediction equation. All references to logs refer to $\log_{10}$.

found to be reliable for general use in the population. The equations of Jackson and Pollock (1978), Jackson et al. (1980) and Durnin and Womersley (1974) will be used (see table 4.5) with the associated skinfold sites identified in table 4.6.

Subjects should be aware that the error in measurement from using skinfolds is about 5 per cent for even a good anthropometrist, and repeated supervised practice is required to reduce the technical error of measurement. Regardless of the method used, there are pre-test conditions that should be adhered to.

Example: Find the predicted % body fat of the following subject using the Durnin and Womersley equation (1974):

Male soccer player, body mass 80kg. Skinfold thicknesses were assessed to be 4.6mm for the biceps, 7mm for the triceps, 6.5mm for subscapular and 14mm for iliac crest (suprailiac).

Step 1 Sum the 4 skinfold thicknesses:

Body density $= 1.1610 - 0.0632\log\sum 4$ sites
Body density $= 1.1610 - 0.0632\log(32.1) = 1.066$

Step 2 Estimate % body fat based on body density using the two equations below, which are the most frequently used and researched.

% body fat $= (4.95/\text{body density} - 4.50) \times 100$ (Siri equation)

% body fat $= (4.57/\text{body density} - 4.142) \times 100$ (Brozek equation)

So predicted % body fat using the Siri equation is:

% body fat $= (4.95/1.066 - 4.50) \times 100$
$= (4.64 - 4.50) \times 100$
$= 14.4$
Therefore body fat $= 14.4\%$

Predicted % body fat using the Brozek equation is:

% body fat $= (4.57/1.066 - 4.142) \times 100$
$= (4.287 - 4.142) \times 100$
$= 14.5$
Therefore body fat $= 14.5\%$

Recommended location of skinfold sites

When identifying specific skinfold sites (irrespective of the test protocol being used, as most sites are common across all methods), testers should follow the ISAK recommendations as shown in table 4.6 related to the precise location of individual sites. The precise location description should help the tester to standardise all repeated measurements and hopefully reduce the tester error as much as possible.

Because of the potential for error with skinfold measurement (especially between different testers), it is important to adhere to pre-test conditions to increase the reliability and reproducibility of measurements.

Table 4.6	ISAK recommended skinfold site locations
Location	Description
Iliac crest	Diagonal/near-horizontal fold raised immediately superior to the crest of the ilium on a vertical line from the mid-axilla. Referred to as the suprailiac by Durnin and Womersley (1974)
Subscapular	Oblique skinfold raised 2cm below and 2cm lateral to the inferior angle of the scapula at ~45° to the horizontal plane following the natural cleavage lines of the skin
Triceps	Vertical skinfold raised on the posterior aspect of the triceps, exactly halfway between the olecranon process and the acromion process. Hand should be supinated
Biceps	Vertical skinfold raised on the anterior aspect of the biceps, at the same horizontal level as the triceps skinfold
Pectoral	Oblique skinfold raised along the border of the pectoralis major, midway between the anterior axillary fold and the nipple in males and a third of the distance in females
Mid-axillary	Vertical skinfold at the mid-axillary line at the level of the xiphoid (lower extremity of the sternum)
Abdominal	Vertical skinfold at 5cm lateral of the midpoint of the umbilicus (belly button)
Mid-thigh	Vertical skinfold raised at the anterior aspect of the thigh, midway between the inguinal crease and the proximal border of the patella when seated with the knee flexed to 90°
Suprailium	Diagonal skinfold above the crest of the ilium at the point where an imaginary line would come down from the anterior axillary border. Slightly anterior to the iliac crest

Pre-test conditions

Ensure that a warm, well-lit room is used and privacy is assured at all times for the subject being tested. If the assessor is male, measurements of females and children should be made sensitively and supervised if possible.

The subject should be relaxed and comfortable (swimsuits – two-piece in the case of women – are ideal although a singlet and shorts may also be suitable).

Subjects should always be clearly informed about the procedures involved in the testing and should be provided with an informed consent form to complete before participation in the test. All measurements should be made on the right-hand side of the body for standardisation purposes.

Required resources

Skinfold calliper, tape measure, marker pen.

Testing method

1. The tester's left hand should raise a skinfold between the thumb and forefinger at the marked site in the required direction, following the natural cleavage lines of the skin (see figure 4.8a).
2. There should be slight rolling and pulling action to separate the fold from the muscle beneath.
3. The calliper is held in the right hand and the blades are applied perpendicularly to the fold and 1cm away from the thumb and forefinger (see figure 4.8b).
4. Spring pressure is released and value is recorded two seconds later to the nearest 0.2 mm.
5. All skinfolds should be measured three times with a two-minute recovery to allow compression of the tissue to return to normal. Measure three times and use the median (middle) value obtained.

| Fig. 4.8a | Grasping a skinfold |

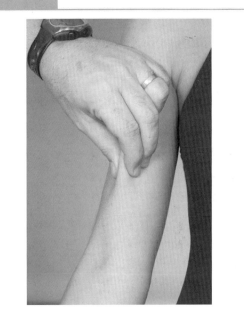

| Fig. 4.8b | Placement of the calliper |

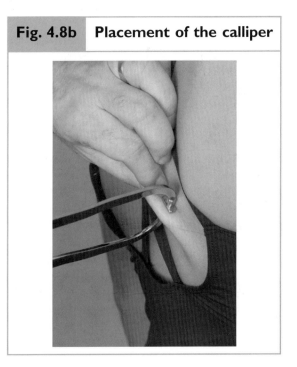

Analysis

Once all of the skinfold sites have been measured (having decided on the method to be used) they should be added together. This sum should then be used for calculation with the relevant equation from table 4.5, depending on the subject being tested. The calculation should then result in an estimation of the subject's body fat percentage.

Alternative analysis

As an alternative to using an equation in table 4.5 to estimate body fat percentage, add up the measurements of all four sites to give a total in millimetres. Find this total millimetre score in the 'Sum' column of table 4.7 and read across to give the body fat percentage. Note that there are age ranges for men and women.

As already discussed within this chapter there are many advantages and disadvantages of methods for assessing body composition depending on the one being used and the individual being tested. Table 4.8 gives a brief summary of both the advantages and disadvantages relating to each method of assessment.

Choice of testing method

As there are many testing methods to choose from, it can be quite confusing deciding how to assess body composition. The following factors should be considered to help in making the choice:

Expense of the equipment

Some equipment used for the measurement of body composition can be relatively expensive, so select within your budget allocation.

Skills or training required

Some equipment requires a greater deal of skill on the part of the tester: therefore a degree of training might be required and this has a cost attached to it. For example, it has been demonstrated in relation to skinfold measurements that the more experienced the tester, the more accurate the measurement is likely to be.

Population to be measured

There are certain methods of testing that would suit certain populations. For example, skinfold callipers are not recommended for obese individuals, as in some cases the size of skinfold can be too large for the calliper. Circumferential methods would then be recommended.

Subject's requirements

Depending on the goals of the individual, it could be the case that a circumferential measurement would suffice (maybe in the case of a client who has a simple weight-loss goal for which size would be a good motivational tool) but, for an athlete who has specific performance targets related to body mass, more sophisticated methods would be necessary.

Time constraints

Some tests are more time consuming than others in relation to delivery and analysis.

Required accuracy of measurement

If the tester and subject require a high degree of accuracy then methods such as underwater weighing and DXA must be considered.

Table 4.7	Skinfold conversion table (Durnin and Womersley)						
	Men (Age in years)				Women (Age in years)		
Sum (mm)	16–29	30–49	>49	Sum (mm)	16–29	30–49	>49
20	8.1	12.1	12.5	14	9.4	14.1	17.0
22	9.2	13.2	13.9	16	11.2	15.7	18.6
24	10.2	14.2	15.1	18	12.7	17.1	20.1
26	11.2	15.2	16.3	20	14.1	18.4	21.4
28	12.1	16.1	17.4	22	15.4	19.5	22.6
30	12.9	16.9	18.5	24	16.5	20.6	23.7
35	14.7	18.7	20.8	26	17.6	21.5	24.8
40	16.3	20.3	22.8	28	18.6	22.4	25.7
45	17.7	21.8	24.7	30	19.5	23.3	26.6
50	19.0	23.0	26.3	35	21.6	25.2	28.6
55	20.2	24.2	27.8	40	23.4	26.8	30.3
60	21.2	25.3	29.1	45	25.0	28.3	31.9
65	22.2	26.3	30.4	50	26.5	29.6	33.2
70	23.2	27.2	31.5	55	27.8	30.8	34.6
75	24.0	28.0	32.6	60	29.1	31.9	35.7
80	24.8	28.8	33.7	65	30.2	32.9	36.7
85	25.6	29.6	34.6	70	31.2	33.9	37.7
90	26.3	30.3	35.5	75	32.2	24.7	38.6
95	27.0	31.0	36.5	80	31.1	25.6	39.5
100	27.6	31.7	37.3	85	34.0	36.3	40.4
110	28.8	32.9	38.8	90	34.8	37.1	41.1
120	29.9	34.0	40.2	95	35.6	37.8	41.9
130	31.1	35.0	41.5	100	36.3	38.5	42.6
140	31.9	36.0	42.8	110	35.7	39.7	43.9
150	32.8	36.8	43.9	120	39.0	40.8	45.1
160	33.6	37.7	45.0	130	4.02	41.9	46.2
170	34.4	38.5	46.0	140	41.3	42.9	47.3
180	35.2	39.2	47.0	150	42.3	43.8	48.2
190	35.9	39.9	47.9	160	43.2	44.7	49.1
200	36.5	40.6	48.8	170	44.6	45.5	50.0

Table 4.8	Advantages and disadvantages of methods for assessing body composition	
Method	**Advantages**	**Disadvantages**
Anthropometry (skinfolds, girths and diameters)	• Relatively inexpensive. • Wide variety of predictive equations for many different populations.	• Requires good technique and site identification. • Difficult to compare between testers. • Measurement errors.
Underwater weighing	• Gold standard for body density. • Forms the basis of many other techniques.	• Need specialised equipment. • Can be uncomfortable. • Difficulty in assessing volumes of trapped gases.
BMI	• Simple to perform. • Linked to health and mortality. • Established norms.	• Limited information on body composition. • Not sensitive for those who are overweight. • Not suitable for many athletic populations.
Waist circumference	• Simple to perform. • Provides information about location of fat deposits most closely linked to health and mortality.	• Limited information about body composition or fat deposits elsewhere on body. • Can be done incorrectly.
Total body water (dilution)	• Simple for subjects to perform. • Used as the basis for bio-impedance.	• Need specialised, expensive equipment. • Greatly affected by diet and hydration status.
Bioimpedance	• Simple for assessors and subjects to perform. • Relatively rapid and non-invasive. • Relatively inexpensive compared to DXA or UW.	• Greatly affected by diet, hydration status and body temperature. • Equations are not always provided by manufacturers.
Near infrared reactance (NIR)	• Simple to use and relatively inexpensive. • Non-invasive and very rapid measurements. • Relatively insensitive to prior diet and hydration.	• Problems associated with assessing body composition based on only one site on the body. • Equations not provided by manufacturers.

Table 4.8	Advantages and disadvantages of methods for assessing body composition (cont.)	
Method	Advantages	Disadvantages
DXA	<ul><li>Becoming the new gold standard for body composition.</li><li>Gives information about fat mass, fat-free mass and bone mass.</li></ul>	<ul><li>Very expensive, specialised equipment and highly trained staff to interpret.</li><li>May be difficult to measure extremely obese individuals on standard size scanners.</li></ul>
BODPOD	<ul><li>Simple to use and relatively inexpensive.</li><li>Non-invasive and relatively rapid measurements.</li></ul>	<ul><li>Very expensive, specialised equipment.</li><li>Potential for error in measuring thoracic gas volumes.</li></ul>

Further reading

American College of Sports Medicine (2002) *ACSM's Exercise Management for Persons with Chronic Diseases and Disabilities*, Champaign, Illinois: Human Kinetics

Arlot, M. E., Sornay-Rendu, E., Garnero, P., Vey-Marty, B. & Delmas, P. D. (1997) 'Apparent pre- and postmenopausal bone loss evaluated by DXA at different skeletal sites in women: The OFELY cohort'. *Journal of Bone Mineral Research*, 12: pp. 683-90

Bakker, H. K. & Struikenkamp, R. S. (1977) 'Biological variability and lean body mass estimates'. *Human Biology*, 53: pp. 181-225

Ball, S. D. & Altena, T. S. (2004) 'Comparison of the BODPOD and dual energy x-ray absorptiometry in men'. *Physiological Measurement*, 25: pp. 671-8

Baumgartner, R. N., Heymsfield, S. B., Lichtman, S., Wang, J. & Pierson, R. N. (1991) 'Body composition in elderly people: Effect of criterion estimates on predictive equations'. *American Journal of Clinical Nutritrion*, 53: pp. 1345-53

Baumgartner, R. N., Rhyne, R. L., Troup, C., Wayne, S. & Garry, P. J. (1992) 'Appendicular skeletal muscle areas assessed by magnetic resonance imaging in older persons'. *Journal of Gerontology*, 47: pp. 67-72

Bjorntorp, P. (1984) 'Hazards in subgroups of human obesity'. *European Journal of Clinical Investigation*, 14: pp. 239-41

Brozek, J., Grande, F., Anderson, J. T. & Keys, A. (1963) 'Densitometric analysis of body composition: Revision of some quantitative assumptions'. *Annals of the New York Academy of Sciences*, 110: pp. 113-140

de Koning, F. L., Binkhorst, R. A., Kauer, J. M. G. & Thijssen, H. O. M. (1986) 'Accuracy of an anthropometric estimate of the muscle and bone area in a transversal cross-section of the arm'. *International Journal of Sports Medicine*, 7: pp. 246-9

Cole, T. J., Freeman, J. V. & Preece, M. A. (1990) 'Body mass index reference curves for the UK'. *British Medical Journal*, 73: pp. 25-9

Drinkwater, D. T., Martin, A. D., Ross, W. D. & Clarys, J. P. (1984) 'Validation by cadaver dissection of Matiegka's equations for the anthropometric estimation of anatomical body composition in adult humans'. In Day, J. A. P. (ed.) *The 1984 Olympic Scientific Congress Proceedings – Perspectives in Kinanthropometry*, Champaign, Illinois: Human Kinetics, pp. 221-7

Durnin, J. V. G. A. & Womersley, J. (1974) 'Body fat assessed from total body density and its estimation from skinfold thickness: Measurements on 481 men and women aged from 16 to 72 years'. *British Journal of Nutrition*, 32: p. 77

Eston, R. G., Kreitzman, S., Lamb, K. L., Brodie, D. A., Robson, S. & Carney, J. (1990) 'Assessment of fat-free mass by hydrodensitometry, skinfolds, infra-red interactance and electrical impedance in boys and girls aged 11–12 years'. *Journal of Sports Sciences*, 8: pp. 174-5

Flegal, K. M., Graubard, B. I., Williamson, D. F. & Gail, M. H. (2005) 'Excess deaths associated with underweight, overweight, and obesity'. *Journal of the American Medical Association*, 293: pp. 1861-7

Fornetti, W. C., Pivarnik, J. M., Foley, J. M. & Fiechtner, J. J. (1999) 'Reliability and validity of body composition measures in female athletes'. *Journal of Applied Physiology*, 87: pp. 1114-22

Garn, S. M., Leonard, W. R. & Hawthorne, V. M. (1986) 'Three limitations of the body mass index'. *American Journal of Clinical Nutrition*, 44: pp. 996-7

Genton, L., Hans, D., Kyle, U. G. & Pichard, C. (2002) 'Dual-energy X-ray absorptiometry and body composition: Differences between devices and comparison with reference methods'. *Nutrition*, 18: pp. 66-70

Gleichauf, C. N. & Roe, D. A. (1989) 'The menstrual cycle's effect on the reliability of bioimpedance measurements for assessing body composition'. *American Journal of Clinical Nutrition*, 50: pp. 903-7

Goldman, R. & Buskirk, E. (1961) 'Body volume measurement by underwater weighing: Description of method'. In Brozek, J. & Henschel, A. (eds.) *Techniques for Measuring Body Composition*, Washington, D. C.: National Academy of Sciences-National Research Council, pp. 78-79

Hawes, M. R. & Sovak, D. (1994) 'Morphological prototypes, assessment and change in young athletes'. *Journal of Sports Sciences*, 12: pp. 235-42

Hawes, M. R. & Martin, A. D. (2001) 'Human body composition'. In Eston, R. G. & Reilly, T. (2001) *Kinanthropometry and Exercise Physiology Laboratory Manual: Tests, Procedures and Data. Volume 1: Anthropometry*, 2nd edn, London, UK: Routledge, pp. 7-46

Heymsfield, S. B., McManus, C., Smith, J., Stevens, V. & Nixon, D. W. (1982). 'Anthropometric measurement of muscle mass: Revised equations for calculating bone-free arm muscle area'. *American Journal of Clinical Nutrition*, 36: pp. 680-90

Heymsfield, S. B., Wang, Z. M. & Withers, R. T. (1996) 'Multi-component molecular level models of body composition analysis'. In Roche, A. F., Heymsfield, S. B. & Lohman, T. G. (eds.) *Human Body Composition*, Champaign, Illinois: Human Kinetics, pp. 129-47

Heyward, V. H. (1996) *Advanced Fitness Assessment and Exercise Prescription*, Champaign, Illinois: Human Kinetics

Hodgdon, J. A. & Fitzgerald, P. I. (1987) 'Validity of impedance predictions at various levels of fatness'. *Human Biology*, 59(2): pp. 281-98

Houtkooper, L. B., Lohman, T. G., Going, S. B. & Hall, M. C. (1989) 'Validity of bioelectrical impedance for body composition assessment in children'. *Journal of Applied Physiology*, 66: pp. 814-21

Houtkooper, L. B., Lohman, T. G., Going, S. B. & Howell, W. H. (1996) 'Why bioelectrical impedance analysis should be used for estimating adiposity'. *American Journal of Clinical Nutrition*, 64(Suppl.): pp. 436S-48S

Jackson, A. S. & Pollock, M. L. (1978) 'Generalized equations for predicting body density in men'. *British Journal of Nutrition*, 40: pp. 497-504

Jackson, A. S., Pollock, M. L. & Ward, A. (1980) 'Generalized equations for predicting body density in women'. *Medicine and Science in Sports and Exercise*, 12: pp. 175-82

Ketel, I. J. G., Volman, N. M., Seidell, J. C., Stehouwer, C. D. A., Twisk, J. W. & Lambalk, C. B. (2007) 'Superiority of skinfold measurements and waist over waist-to-hip ratio for determination of body fat distribution in a population-based cohort of Caucasian Dutch adults'. *European Journal of Endocrinology*, 156(6), pp. 655-61

Kohrt, W. M. (1995) 'Body composition by DXA: Tried and true?'. *Medicine and Science in Sports and Exercise*, 27: pp. 1349-53

Kushner, R. F. (1992) 'Bioelectrical impedance analysis: A review of principles and applications'. *Journal of the American College of Nutrition*, 11: pp. 199-209

Lohman, T. G. (1981) 'Skinfold and body density and their relationship to body fatness: A review'. *Human Biology*, 53: pp. 181-225

Lohman, T. G., Slaughter, M. H., Boileau, R. A., Bunt, J. & Lussier, L. (1984) 'Bone mineral measurements and their relation to body density in children, youth and adults'. *Human Biology*, 56: pp. 667-9

Lohman, T. G. (1992) *Advances in body composition assessment. Current issues in exercise science series* (Monograph 3), Champaign, Illinois: Human Kinetics

Lukaski, H. C., Bolonchuk, W. W., Hall, C. B., Siders, W. A. (1986) 'Validation of tretrapolar bioelectric impedance method to assess human body composition'. *Journal of Applied Physiology*, 60: pp. 1327-32

Lukaski, H. C. (1987) 'Methods for the assessment of human composition: Traditional and new'. *American Journal of Clinical Nutrition*, 46: pp. 537-56

Martin, A. D., Ross, W. D., Drinkwater, D. T. & Clarys, J. P. (1985) 'Prediction of body fat by skinfold caliper: Assumptions and cadaver evidence'. *International Journal of Obesity*, 9: pp. 31-9

Martin, A. D., Drinkwater, D. T., Clarys, J. P. & Ross, W. D. (1986) 'The inconstancy of the fat-free mass: A reappraisal with applications for densitometry'. In Reilly, T. J. (ed.) *Kinanthropometry III. Proceedings of the VII Commonwealth and International Conference on Sport, Physical Education, Dance, Recreation and Health*, London, UK: E & FN Spon, pp. 92-7

Martin, A. D., Spenst, L. F., Drinkwater, D. T. & Clarys, J. P. (1990) 'Anthropometric estimation of muscle mass in men'. *Medicine and Science in Sports and Exercise*, 22: pp. 729-33

Martin, A. D., Drinkwater, D. T., Clarys, J. P., Daniel, M. & Ross, W. D. (1992) 'Effects of skin thickness and skinfold compressibility on skinfold thickness measurement'. *American Journal of Human Biology*, 6: pp. 1-8

Martin, A. D. & Drinkwater, D. T. (1991) 'Variability in the measures of body fat'. *Sports Medicine*, 11: pp. 277-88

Mast, M., Langnase, K., Labitzke, K., Bruse, U., Preub, U. & Muller, M. J. (2002) 'Use of BMI as a measure of overweight and obesity in a field study on 5–7-year-old children'. *European Journal of Nutrition*, 41: pp. 61-7

Miller, W. C., Swenson, T. & Wallace, J. P. (1998) 'Derivation of prediction equations for RV in overweight men and women'. *Medicine and Science in Sport and Exercise*, 30: pp. 322-7

Moon, J. R., Hull, H. R., Tobkin, S. E., Teramoto, M., Karabulut, M., Roberts, M. D., Ryan, E. D., Kim, S. J., Dalbo, V. J., Walter, A. A., Smith, A. E., Cramer, J. T. & Stout, J. R. (2007) 'Percent body fat estimations in college women using field and laboratory methods: A three-compartment model approach'. *Journal of the International Society of Sports Nutrition*, 4: p. 16

National Institute for Health and Clinical Excellence (2006) 'Obesity: The prevention, identification, assessment and management of overweight and obesity in adults and children'. London, UK: NICE

Nyboar, J., Bagno, S. & Nims, L. F. (1943) 'The electrical impedance plethysmograph and electrical volume recorder'. Washington, D. C.: National Research Council, Committee on Aviation

Price, G. M., Uauy, R., Breeze, E., Bulpitt, C. J. & Fletcher, A. E. (2006) 'Weight, shape, and mortality risk in older persons: Elevated waist-hip ratio, not high body mass index, is associated with a greater risk of death'. *American Journal of Clinical Nutrition*, 84: pp. 449-60

Prior, B. M., Modlesky, C. M., Evans, E. M., Sloniger, M. A., Saunders, M. A., Lewis, R. J. & Cureton, K. J. (2001). 'Muscularity and the density of the fat-free mass in athletes'. *Journal of Applied Physiology*, 90: pp. 1523–31

Ross, W. D., Eiben, O. G., Ward, R., Martin, A. D., Drinkwater, D. T. & Clarys, J. P. (1986) 'Alternatives for conventional methods of human body composition and physique assessment'. In Day, J. A. P. (ed.) *The 1984 Olympic Scientific Congress Proceedings – Perspectives in Kinanthropometry*, Champaign, Illinois: Human Kinetics, pp. 203-20

Ross, W. D., Martin, A. D. & Ward, R. (1987) 'Body composition and aging: Theoretical and methodological implications'. *Coll. Anthropometry*, 11: pp. 15-44

Segal, K. R., van Loan, M., Fitzgerald, P. I., Hodgson, J. A. & Van Itallie, T. B. (1988) 'Lean body mass estimation by bioelectrical impedance analysis: A four-site cross-validation study'. *American Journal of Clinical Nutrition*, 47: pp. 7-14

Sheng, H. P. & Huggins, R. A. (1979) 'A review of body composition studies with emphasis on total body water and fat'. *American Journal of Clinical Nutrition*, 32: pp. 630-47

Siri, W. E. (1956) 'Body composition from fluid spaces and density: Analysis of methods'. University of California Radiation Laboratory, Report UCRL no. 3349

van Loan, M. D. & Mayclin, P. (1987) 'Bioelectrical impedance analysis: Is it a reliable estimator of lean body mass and total body water?' *Human Biology*, 59: pp. 299-309

van Loan, M. D. (1990) 'Bioelectrical impedance analysis to determine fat-free mass, total body water and body fat'. *Sports Medicine*, 10(4): pp. 205-17

von Eyben, F. E., Mouritsen, E., Holm, J., Montvilas, P., Dimcevski, G., Suciu, G. P. (2006) 'Computed tomography scans of intra-abdominal fat, anthropometric measurements, and three non-obese metabolic risk factors'. *Metabolism: Clinical and Experimental*, 55: pp. 1337-43

Wang, Z. M., Pierson, R. N., Jr. & Heymsfield, S. B. (1992) 'The five-level model: A new approach to organizing body composition research'. *American Journal of Clinical Nutrition*, 56: pp. 19-28

Ward, A., Pollock, M. L., Jackson, A. S., Ayres, J. J. & Pape, G. (1978) 'A comparison of body fat determined by underwater weighing and volume displacement'. *American Journal of Physiology*, 234: pp. E94-E96

Wei, M., Gaskill, S. P., Haffner, S. M. & Stern, M. P. (1997) 'Waist circumference as the best predictor of noninsulin dependent diabetes mellitus (NIDDM) compared to body mass index, waist/hip ratio, and other anthropometric measurements in Mexican Americans – A 7-year prospective study'. *Obesity Research*, 5: pp. 16-23

Wilmore, J. H. & Behnke, A. R. (1969) 'An anthropometric estimation of body density and lean body weight in young men'. *Journal of Applied Physiology*, 27: pp. 25-31

Withers, R. T., LaForgia, J., Pillans, R. K., Shipp, N. J., Chatterton, B. E., Schultz, C. G. & Leaney, F. (1998) 'Comparisons of two-, three-, and four-compartment models of body composition analysis in men and women'. *Journal of Applied Physiology*, 85: pp. 238–45

FLEXIBILITY TESTING

5

OBJECTIVES

After completing this chapter you should be able to:

1 Define what is meant by the term 'flexibility' and explain the difference between static and dynamic forms.

2 Explain the terms 'static', 'dynamic', 'ballistic' and 'PNF' stretching in relation to range of motion.

3 Explain the stretch reflex mechanism and its effect on stretching.

4 List and discuss the types of joint range of motion constraints that can limit flexibility.

5 List and explain the different physiological and neural factors that contribute to joint stability.

6 Describe the difference between, and give examples of, direct and indirect methods of assessing flexibility.

7 List and describe the common methods of testing for joint range of motion.

8 Identify common body landmarks for goniometer assessment purposes.

9 List and describe a range of typical goniometer tests for specific joints in the body.

10 List and describe a range of typical adapted range of motion tests for various populations.

Flexibility

Flexibility is usually associated with the range of motion (ROM) around joints in the body, and this allows individuals to carry out daily activities as long as possible throughout their lives. Flexibility can also be thought of in dynamic (motion-related) terms, for example how compliant the muscles are in allowing a joint to go through its full range of motion without any stiffness or resistance to that movement. There are many types of stretching exercise, including static and dynamic, and also ballistic and PNF which are considered to increase both types of flexibility.

Types of stretching exercise

Static

When a stretch is performed and held for a period of time at a point of mild tension it is known as a static stretch. The point of tension is usually the point at which the stretch reflex is invoked. If the stretch is held long enough, this tension usually subsides and the stretch can be taken further if required. If a partner or another group of muscles assists in the stretching process it is called an *active* stretch. If there is no assistance in the stretch it is called a *passive* stretch. Research on the optimum time period for a stretch is vague.

Dynamic

This term relates to stretching in motion where an agonist muscle is contracted to stretch an antagonist muscle. This type of stretching is usually carried out in a slow and controlled

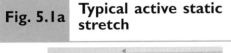

Fig. 5.1a Typical active static stretch

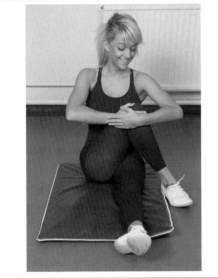

Fig. 5.1b Typical passive static stretch

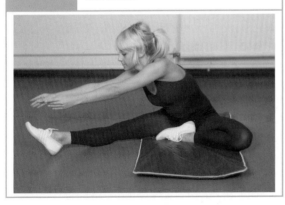

manner in order to minimise the risk of injury and to mimic the types of movement that may be used in the exercises to follow. This has been described as 'the ability to use a range of joint movement in the performance of a physical activity at normal or rapid speed' (Alter 1996). Alter suggests that this type of flexibility is more

Fig. 5.2 Typical dynamic stretch

applicable to sports-specific exercise as it involves movement, as opposed to static flexibility, which does not.

Ballistic

This involves bouncing movements caused by momentum or gravity. It is usually carried out by athletes who are familiar with this type of stretching. As there is little control of the movement there is a greater risk of injury.

PNF

Proprioceptive neuromuscular facilitation (PNF) is a type of partner-assisted stretching, usually of tight or injured muscles. There is usually a degree of training associated with this type of stretching, so it should be performed only by those who are qualified to do so. CRAC (Contract, Relax, Antagonist, Contract) is another form of this type of stretching.

It is widely accepted that both static and dynamic flexibility are an important integral

Fig. 5.3	**Typical ballistic stretch**

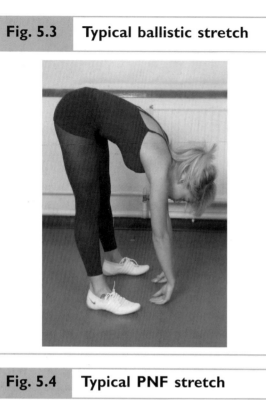

Fig. 5.4	**Typical PNF stretch**

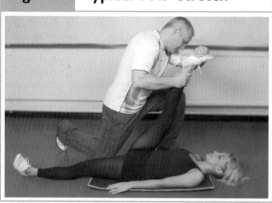

part of any training routine; however, many authors suggest that it is the warmth of the muscle that is the most important factor in reducing the risk of injury, as opposed to the common perception that it is the stretching.

There appears to be no general consensus of prescription for flexibility exercises, and no conclusive statements have been made about the relationship of flexibility to injury, as many research studies report opposing findings. It is worth noting that the European College of Sports Sciences states the following:

'. . . data overwhelmingly appears to refute the notion that stretching exercise influences the resistance to stretch in the long term . . . and it is tolerance to stretch that appears to affect short-term gains.'

In relation to performing various types of stretching exercise, the speed of the stretch is important due to the nature of the mechanism known as the *stretch reflex*.

Stretch reflex

One of the most important structures that contribute to the stretch reflex is that of the *muscle spindle*. Otherwise known as an *intrafusal fibre*, this is simply a modified muscle fibre that is usually found in parallel to a normal muscle fibre (which is known as an *extrafusal fibre*).

When muscle fibres change their length as in stretching, the muscle spindles also change their length correspondingly, as they lie in parallel. Muscle spindles contain two types of fibre, termed *bag* and *chain* fibres. These names refer to the distribution of nuclei within a fibre (in either a bag or a chain configuration).

Bag fibres come in two types, static and dynamic. Sensory endings called *primary spindle endings* are located mostly in the middle portion of the spindle and sense both muscle length and velocity of stretch of the muscle. The frequency of firing of the primary spindle ending is thought to be higher after a stretch than before, which indicates that the ending is sensitive to muscle *length*. The frequency of firing of the ending is also higher for faster stretches, which means that the ending is sensitive to the *velocity* of the stretch as well.

There are implications of these responses

relevant to both static-type (slow) stretches and dynamic movement-type (fast) stretches employed in many sports and vigorous activities. For example, faster stretches carried out in any muscle fibres will initiate a more powerful contraction of the muscle being stretched, due to the reflex response (the stretch reflex as it is known) of the action potentials from the primary endings of the muscle spindles. In other words, the faster a muscle is stretched, the more powerful it will try to contract against the stretch, as can be seen in figure 5.5. For this reason it is recommended that static-type stretches be carried out at slow stretch speeds to minimise the reaction of the stretch reflex system.

The length of the muscle fibres being stretched also determines the contribution of the stretch reflex system. The more a muscle is stretched, the greater the contraction within the muscle as a result of the stretch reflex system. It is recommended that stretches should be taken only to the point of mild tension.

Those individuals with tighter than normal muscles would probably benefit most from stretching, whereas those individuals who have naturally supple muscle tissue should not engage in more than light stretching. One of the main reasons for this is that, as commonly agreed, the muscular system (muscle and its fascia) is one of the three main systems that can make an important contribution to joint stability. It should also be remembered that the most effective stretching (from an improvement perspective) normally occurs when the muscles are thoroughly warm.

As far as testing is concerned, flexibility should also be considered as joint specific, in that an individual may be flexible in one joint but not necessarily flexible in others. Therefore, when testing for joint flexibility, the tester should be aware that there is no single test that could be defined as a whole-body flexibility test. In order to achieve this, all joints of the body must be assessed for flexibility on an individual basis. There are certain physiological constraints that can affect flexibility, or joint range of motion as it is more accurately termed.

Constraints on joint range of motion can be broadly classified in two distinct groups, *active constraints* and *passive constraints*. The main components of active constraints include muscle and tendon tissue, whereas the main components of passive constraints include bone, joint capsule, ligaments and cartilage. Muscle is composed of more elastic tissue than structures such as the joint capsule, ligaments and tendons; therefore, it is probably the most easily modifiable constraint in terms of increasing range of joint motion.

Fig. 5.5   Stretch reflex

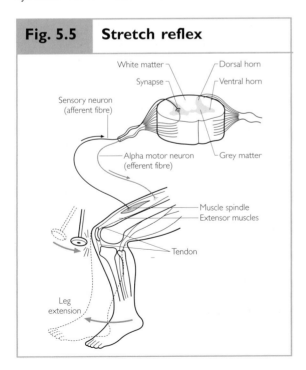

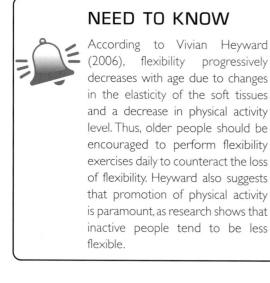

NEED TO KNOW

According to Vivian Heyward (2006), flexibility progressively decreases with age due to changes in the elasticity of the soft tissues and a decrease in physical activity level. Thus, older people should be encouraged to perform flexibility exercises daily to counteract the loss of flexibility. Heyward also suggests that promotion of physical activity is paramount, as research shows that inactive people tend to be less flexible.

Although not considered to be a modifiable constraint, the configuration of joints can play an important role in determining their range of motion. For instance, the shoulder joint (humerus, scapula and clavicle) is much more flexible than the hip joint (femur and pelvis) because, even though they are both 'ball and socket' synovial joints, the hip joint is much deeper than the shoulder joint. This is because the hip joint requires far greater stability for everyday use, and the shoulder joint requires a greater range of motion. As flexibility requirements also differ greatly depending on the sport, event or everyday need of the subject being tested, much thought should be given by the tester to the degree of flexibility required in relation to specific joint range of motion.

Joint stability

Flexibility beyond a 'normal' range of motion may be useful or necessary for the performance of certain sports or specific event skills but, for the purpose of joint stability, remember that the muscular system is considered to be one of the main systems that can make an important contribution to the potential prevention of injury.

The three main systems that are generally considered to contribute to overall joint stability are shown in figure 5.6. All three are widely accepted to be of major importance in the prevention of injury mainly as a result of joint laxity or instability. Ligament tissue is prone to tears, rupture and deformation: therefore, the muscular system is often required to provide a greater amount of stability for joints, especially during dynamic movements. In many cases, where the flexibility of an individual is considered to be beyond the normal range of motion (often referred to as hyper-flexibility), joint stability is often lacking or reduced. This can result in a variety of conditions of joint injury. In cases where the flexibility of an individual is considered to be less than the normal range, injury such as muscle strain can occur.

Normal ranges of motion at specific joints have been published by bodies such as the American College of Sports Medicine and the American Medical Association (AMA).

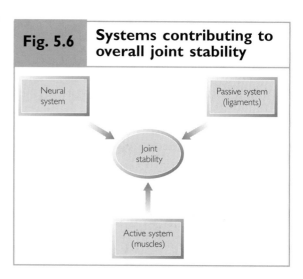

Fig. 5.6 **Systems contributing to overall joint stability**

Assessment of flexibility

There are several laboratory and field-based assessment techniques that have been developed for assessing flexibility. However, most of these methods are for measurements of static flexibility, as little research has been done on the assessment of dynamic flexibility (see earlier description of static and dynamic flexibility on page 92). For athletes, most movements are dynamic rather than static and hence dynamic flexibility is more relevant than static flexibility. However, it is more difficult to measure dynamic flexibility than static flexibility and thus it is not commonly measured.

Access to a digital camera/video and some simple measurement software would allow measurement of dynamic flexibility. More advanced software, such as Dartfish, would allow for more sophisticated analysis of flexibility. Dynamic flexibility can be measured by positioning markers at anatomical landmarks and measuring angles during dynamic movements (see figure 5.7).

| Fig. 5.7 | **Positioning markers for the Dartfish system** |

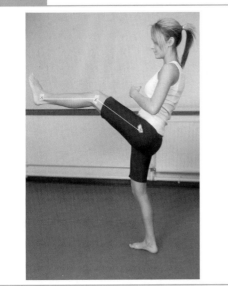

These markers are best placed physically on the subject, but may be added 'virtually' during video analysis.

Dynamic flexibility is affected by the strength of the muscle groups involved in the movement (i.e. both the agonist and antagonist muscles). There are few norms for dynamic flexibility, due to the wide variety of methods by which it is measured.

Static flexibility on the other hand is a parameter that is often overlooked by coaches and instructors but it can be easily measured by using either *direct* or *indirect* methods. A direct method is usually considered to involve angular measures of single joints, whereas indirect methods involve linear measurements.

One of the most common direct methods of measuring static flexibility or range of motion is by a technique known as *goniometry*, in which either electrical or manual goniometer devices are used to measure individual joint angles. This type of direct flexibility testing is considered to be a reasonably valid method of assessment as long as the tester is experienced in using the type of goniometer device needed.

In relation to indirect techniques, there are several methods of assessing flexibility; the *sit-and-reach* test and its modified version are probably the most common field-based methods of assessment used by coaches and instructors. It is cheap and easy to administer as well as being considered a reasonably valid measurement (although this is often argued) for certain subject groups.

NEED TO KNOW

The term 'goniometry' comes from the Greek words 'gonia' meaning angle and 'metron' meaning measure!

Goniometry

The type of flexibility testing known as goniometry is a specific technique used where the angle of each joint (or of specific joints, depending on the requirements of the subject) is measured. The results acquired are then compared against data tables for normal ranges of motion. This type of testing is normally carried out by clinically trained and experienced individuals, with a view to analysing the restricted movement of subjects with lifestyle issues, or of athletes with specific sport or event requirements.

Goniometers are capable of measuring static positions of limb segments with respect to the range of motion (ROM) available at a specific joint. The ROM of a joint refers to the number of degrees through which it is capable of moving.

The goniometer is based on the protractor concept, where one arm is fixed at zero degrees and the other arm is extended from the centre of the protractor and is free to rotate. It can therefore calculate the angle of the joint being measured. The angle of the joint is taken from the insertion of the freely rotating arm and measured on the protractor scale.

Remember, the range of motion is joint and individual specific, and the requirement for a particular joint range of motion is related to the lifestyle or sport demands of the subject being tested. However, for the purpose of testing for subjects who are interested in maintaining quality of life, table 5.1 provides a general overview of typical range of motion values (measured in degrees) that are related to specific joints in the body. The lower value in the range represents the point at which there is possible impairment to the joint.

Table 5.1	Typical ROM values for specific joints	
Joint	Movement pattern	Expected range of motion (degrees)
Shoulder	Flexion	160–170
Shoulder	Extension	40–62
Shoulder	Internal rotation	60–70
Shoulder	External rotation	60–104
Hip	Flexion	90–155
Hip	Extension	9–29
Hip	Internal rotation	26–50
Hip	External rotation	26–70
Hip	Abduction	30–40
Hip	Adduction	10–30
Knee	Flexion	140–145
Knee	Extension	0–5
Ankle	Dorsiflexion	10–20
Ankle	Plantarflexion	30–50

Fig. 5.8	**Typical goniometer**

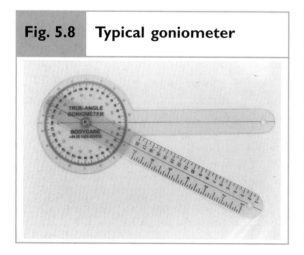

When testing range of motion by goniometry, the device must be placed accurately each time so that results are reliable. The goniometer should be placed so that the centre of the device (where the two arms meet) coincides with the fulcrum or pivot of the specific joint being measured. The joint fulcrums are known as goniometer landmarks and are precise in their description. The range of motion is taken as the difference (measured in degrees) between the two arms of the goniometer at the extremes of the movement related to the specific joint.

There are several types of device available for measuring joint angles. One such device is an *inclinometer*, which is otherwise often referred to as a clinical goniometer. Essentially, the inclinometer is a device with a 360° dial that can be rotated on its own mount and is capable of measuring joint angles in a similar way to the goniometer.

Several problems have been identified in relation to the reliability of goniometer joint-angle measuring. One is the potential difficulty for the investigator in identifying the axis of motion and goniometer placement. This problem can occur at several joints, depending on the experience of the investigator.

The investigator should ideally possess good skills in being able to palpate (feel) the subject in order to identify the precise location of each landmark related to the specific joint. Table 5.2 describes (in anatomical terms) the precise location of common landmarks that should be used

Table 5.2	Common landmarks for goniometry	
Joint	Sagittal plane	Frontal plane
Wrist	Midway between the anterior/posterior surfaces on the distal wrist crease.	Junction of the palmaris longus tendon and the distal wrist crease.
Elbow	On a line through the humeral epicondyles at 1cm proximal to the head of the radius.	At mid-point of a line through the humeral epicondyles at 1cm proximal to the head of the radius.
Shoulder	Midway between the anterior/posterior surfaces at 5cm inferior to the acromion process.	On a vertical line 5cm inferior to the acromion process.
Trunk	Base of the last rib in line with the greater trochanter.	N/A
Hip	Lateral point of the greater trochanter at 3cm superior and 1cm anteriorly.	Horizontal projection to the skin crease at the top of the leg.
Knee	Mid-point of a line through the centres of the posterior convexities of the femoral condyles.	Mid-point of the medial and lateral femoral condyles.
Ankle	Most distal palpable point of the lateral malleolus.	Horizontal projection midway between the lateral and medial surfaces posteriorly.

when performing goniometer measurements. It is also recommended, for reliability purposes, that, when taking a reading from the goniometer, the investigator reads the device at eye level. This is done in order to prevent, or at least minimise, the errors associated with reading the goniometer scale. It is also important that the same device and the same time of day should be used for groups of subjects or repeat testing. It is important to try to standardise the test protocol, as there are many research studies that have established the reliability of this type of direct testing.

The methods for taking goniometer measurements described later in this chapter refer to the *end point* of the range of motion of a joint. This term refers to the end of the range of motion at a particular joint, in a particular plane of motion, before active or passive constraints restrict the movement further without excessive pressure. It is important to note, however, that care should be taken to move the limb slowly towards this point to avoid any risk of potential damage to the joint structures. It may be necessary, though, to apply slight pressure on the joint at this end point, but no excessive pressure should be used.

Because of the required accuracy in testing of this kind, there is a great deal of skill involved on the part of the tester in the measurement technique, not just in the identification of the landmarks but for the placement and reading of the device itself. It is recommended, therefore, that before undertaking goniometer measuring, testers should undergo a period of shadow-training with a competent and qualified supervisor. This period of training should help the tester to identify the landmark points and become familiar with the device, which should subsequently reduce the potential errors associated with this type of measurement technique.

It is also important that, whenever a subject is tested for flexibility, a pre-test warm-up should be carried out in order to fully warm the muscles that are to be tested. The warm-up should be a standardised protocol that can be reproduced in order to maintain the reproducibility of the test. It is also common that subjects are then allowed to perform pre-test stretches of the muscles to be tested. Again, this should be standardised for reproducibility purposes. Care should be taken by the tester to avoid testing in a cold environment because, if the test takes more than a few minutes, there is a possibility that the muscle temperature of the subject being tested may drop and affect the accuracy of the measurement to follow.

With all joint testing it is common for three measurements to be taken and the greatest angle recorded.

As goniometer equipment is not always available, there are several adapted range of motion tests that are described in this chapter. Adapted tests require only a tape measure or measuring stick to measure range of motion.

One of the main disadvantages of this type of adapted testing is that there is a limited range of normative value tables for comparison purposes. If testers choose to use this type of testing, then the results of the subject should be used as a baseline measurement to compare against subsequent range of motion tests.

Goniometer testing methods

The amount of research relating to goniometer and associated adapted testing methods is vast. The methods identified here, and the associated range of motion normative values, are based on a selection of that research and adapted for the benefit of the coach or instructor with ease of implementation and evaluation in mind. You should be aware, however, that there are many other suggested goniometer and adapted testing methods relating to each individual joint in the body. Therefore, you should try to identify and become familiar with a wide range of published methods so that the choice of the testing method to be used is specific to the subject's sport, event or lifestyle demands (and indeed their goals).

The following descriptions (protocols) of commonly used goniometer and adapted joint range of motion measurement methods are considered to be for general flexibility and lifestyle purposes and therefore not necessarily related to any particular sport or event, although they might be chosen in a specific sports context.

The protocol for pre-test warm-up and pre-stretch should also take into consideration the type of subject being tested. Both the warm-up and the pre-stretch protocol should be related to the associated sport of the subject, or should be suitable for general lifestyle purposes should the subject just require general flexibility. There are many published articles (some referenced at the end of this chapter) where warm-up and pre-stretch protocols, related to specific subject groups and specific joint range of motion testing, can be found.

Shoulder flexion

1. The subject stands upright on the floor with both arms by the side of the body.
2. The tester lifts one arm upwards and towards the front of the body (shoulder flexion) until the end point.
3. Slight pressure should be maintained at this point.
4. Measure the angle from the vertical to the line between the landmark points in the sagittal plane for the shoulder and elbow.
5. Repeat for the other arm.

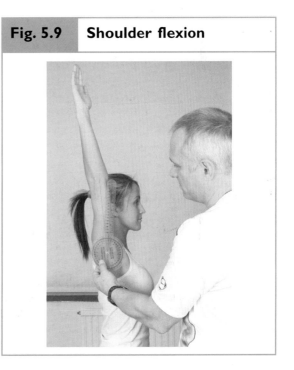

Fig. 5.9 **Shoulder flexion**

Fig. 5.10	Shoulder extension

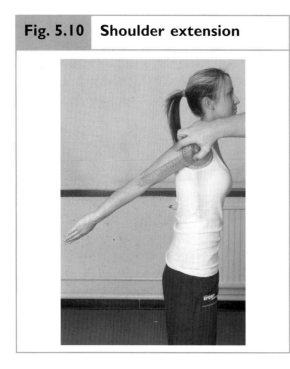

Shoulder extension

1. The subject stands upright on the floor with both arms by the side of the body.
2. The tester lifts one arm upwards and towards the rear of the body (shoulder extension) until the end point (figure 5.10).
3. Slight pressure should be maintained at this point.
4. Measure the angle from the vertical to the line between the landmark points in the sagittal plane for the shoulder and elbow.
5. Repeat for the other arm.

Shoulder internal rotation

1. The subject lies supine with both legs on the couch and one arm by the side.
2. The tester places the other arm so that the upper arm is at 90° to the body and the elbow joint is also at 90° with the forearm vertical (figure 5.11a).
3. The tester rotates the upper arm by bringing the lower arm towards the floor (in the direction of the lower body) until the end point (figure 5.11b).
4. Measure the angle from the vertical to the line between the landmark points in the sagittal plane for the elbow and wrist.
5. Repeat for the other arm.

Shoulder external rotation

1. The subject lies supine with both legs on the couch and one arm by the side.
2. The tester places the other arm so that the upper arm is at 90° to the body and the elbow joint is also at 90° with the forearm vertical (figure 5.12a).
3. The tester rotates the upper arm by bringing the lower arm towards the floor (in the direction of the upper body) until the end point (figure 5.12b).
4. Measure the angle from the vertical to the line between the landmark points in the sagittal plane for the elbow and wrist.
5. Repeat for the other arm.

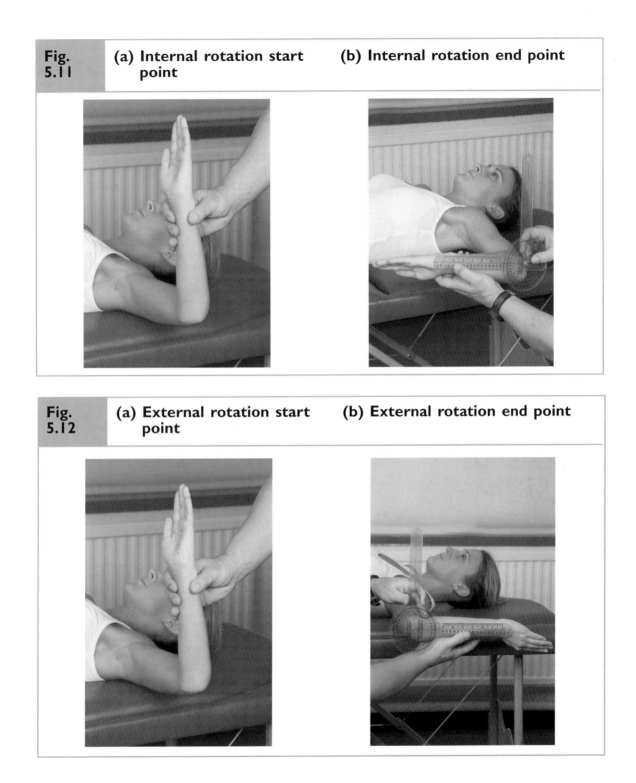

Fig. 5.11

(a) Internal rotation start point

(b) Internal rotation end point

Fig. 5.12

(a) External rotation start point

(b) External rotation end point

Hip flexion

1. The subject lies supine with both legs on the couch and maintains neutral spine throughout.
2. The tester raises one leg (hip flexion), with the thigh towards the torso and the knee joint in flexion.
3. Stop at the end-point.
4. Measure the angle from the horizontal to the line between the hip and knee landmarks in the sagittal plane.
5. Repeat for the other leg.

Hip extension

1. The subject stands at the end of the couch and leans over to support torso on the couch.
2. The non-supporting leg is raised in extension and supported by the tester.
3. Stop at the end point.
4. Measure the angle from the horizontal to the line between the hip and knee landmark points in the sagittal plane.
5. Repeat for the other leg.

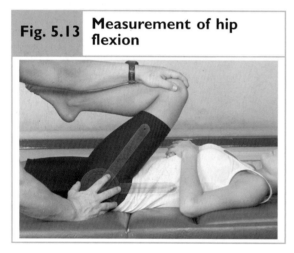

Fig. 5.13 **Measurement of hip flexion**

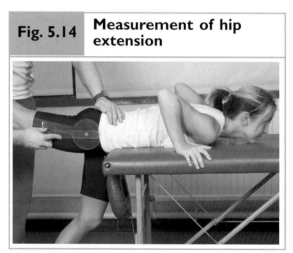

Fig. 5.14 **Measurement of hip extension**

Hip internal rotation

1. The subject lies prone on the couch with knees bent to 90°.
2. The tester rotates the lower leg outward to the end-stop, ensuring that the pelvis remains on the couch at all times.
3. The upper leg should be rotating from the hip.
4. Measure the angle from the vertical line to the line between the landmark points in the frontal plane at the knee and ankle.
5. Repeat for the other leg.

Hip external rotation

1. The subject lies prone on the couch with one leg straight and the other knee bent to 90°.
2. The tester rotates the lower flexed leg inward to the end-stop, ensuring that the pelvis remains on the couch at all times.
3. The upper leg should be rotating from the hip.
4. Measure from the vertical line to the line between the landmark points in the frontal plane at the knee and ankle.
5. Repeat for the other leg.

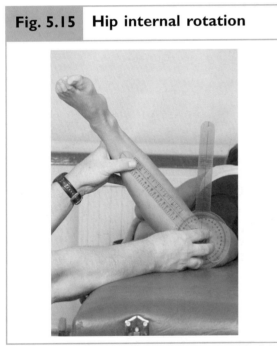

Fig. 5.15 Hip internal rotation

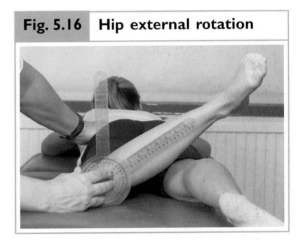

Fig. 5.16 Hip external rotation

Hip abduction

1. The subject lies supine on the couch and maintains neutral spine throughout.
2. Without rotating the leg, the tester abducts the whole leg to the end stop.
3. The leg should be moving from the hip joint.
4. Measure the angle from the neutral line to the line between the landmark points in the frontal plane for the hip and knee.
5. Repeat for the other leg.

Hip adduction

1. The subject lies supine on the couch and maintains neutral spine throughout.
2. Without rotating the leg, the tester lifts the whole leg off the couch and adducts the whole leg to the end stop.
3. The leg should be moving from the hip joint.
4. Measure the angle from the neutral line to the line between the landmark points in the frontal plane for the hip and knee.
5. Repeat for the other leg.

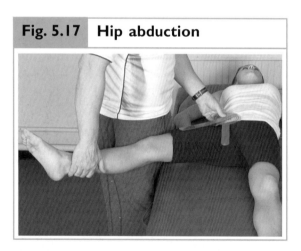

Fig. 5.17 **Hip abduction**

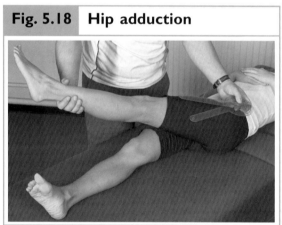

Fig. 5.18 **Hip adduction**

Knee extension

1. The subject lies supine on the couch with both legs out straight and maintains neutral spine throughout.
2. The tester places one hand on the thigh just above the knee joint and the other hand under the leg just above the ankle joint.
3. From this position with slight pressure, pull the lower leg into extension with slight pressure until the end point.
4. Measure the angle from the horizontal line to the line between the landmark points in the sagittal plane for the knee and ankle.
5. Repeat for the other leg.

Knee flexion

1. The subject lies prone on the couch and maintains neutral spine throughout with the hips remaining on the couch at all times.
2. The tester lifts the lower leg into flexion with slight pressure until the end point.
3. Measure the angle from the horizontal line to the line between the landmark points in the sagittal plane for the knee and ankle.
4. Repeat for the other leg.

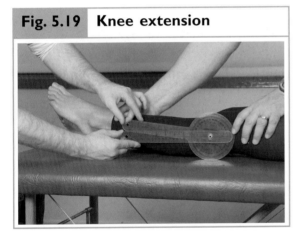

Fig. 5.19 | **Knee extension**

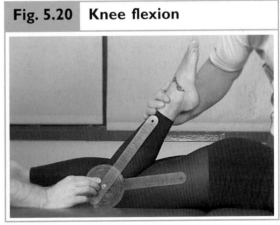

Fig. 5.20 | **Knee flexion**

Ankle plantarflexion

1. The subject lies supine or sits on the couch with the legs out straight.
2. The tester should apply slight pressure on the foot to take the ankle joint to the end point of plantarflexion.
3. Measure the angle from the horizontal line to the line between the landmarks in the sagittal plane of the knee and ankle.
4. Only slight pressure should be applied at the end point and repeat for the other leg.

Ankle dorsiflexion

1. The subject lies supine or sits on the couch with legs out straight.
2. The tester should apply slight pressure on the foot to take the ankle joint to the end point of dorsiflexion.
3. Measure the angle from the horizontal line to the line between the landmarks in the sagittal plane of the knee and ankle.
4. Only slight pressure should be applied at the end point and repeat for the other leg.

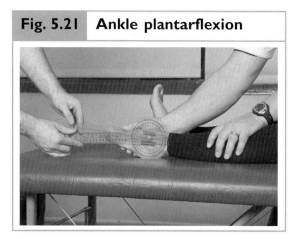

Fig. 5.21 **Ankle plantarflexion**

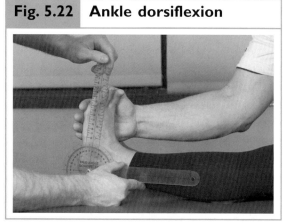

Fig. 5.22 **Ankle dorsiflexion**

Adapted tests with normative data

If goniometer devices are not available then typical measurements can be made using either a measuring stick or tape measure to determine joint flexibility. This type of adapted testing will, however, be prone to greater errors than goniometer testing.

Lumbar extension

1. The subject lies prone on the floor with arms at the sides.
2. The feet should be kept together with toes on the ground.
3. The subject raises the chest off the floor as high as possible.
4. Measure the distance from the nose to the floor.
5. Subtract this measurement from the distance between the nose and the seat of a chair when sitting erect.

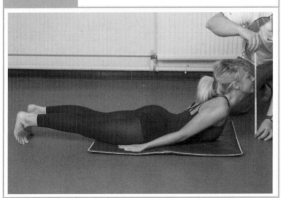

Fig. 5.23   **Lumbar extension**

Ankle plantarflexion

1. The subject sits on the floor with one leg out straight and the foot in the neutral position.
2. Measure the distance from the floor to the lowest point of the tibia (figure 5.24a).
3. Extend the ankle as far as possible.
4. Measure the distance from the floor to the highest point on the dorsal surface of the foot (figure 5.24b).
5. Record the difference between the two measurements.

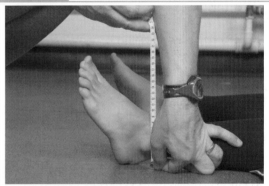

Fig. 5.24a   **Ankle plantarflexion start**

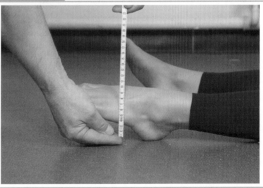

Fig. 5.24b   **Ankle plantarflexion finish**

Ankle dorsiflexion

1. The subject faces a wall standing about 30cm away from the base.
2. The subject then leans forward to touch the wall with hands, chin and chest.
3. The subject must then try to develop as much distance as possible between the wall and the heels, but the heels must remain on the floor at all times.
4. The hands, chest and chin must also remain on the wall.
5. Measure the greatest distance between the toes and the wall.
6. Subtract this measurement from the distance between the floor and the subject's chin while standing upright.

Analysis

The measurements recorded could be used as baseline test data and subsequent test measurements could therefore be used for comparison for either improvement or deterioration of specific joint flexibility.

Classification

Although there are few published normative data tables for this type of testing, table 5.3 could be used as a general classification guide.

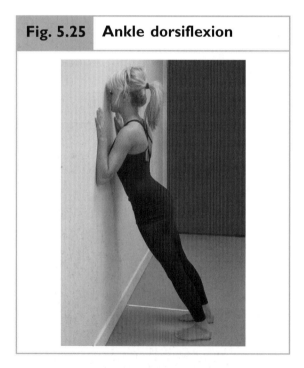

Fig. 5.25 Ankle dorsiflexion

Table 5.3	General flexibility ranges for adapted tests		
	Rating	Men	Women
Lumbar extension	Excellent	3.0 or less	2.0 or less
	Good	6.0–3.25	5.75–2.25
	Average	8.0–6.25	7.75–6.0
	Fair	10.0–8.25	9.75–8.0
	Poor	10.25 or more	10.0 or more
Ankle plantarflexion	Excellent	0.75 or less	0.5 or less
	Good	1.5–1.0	1.25–0.75
	Average	2.0–1.75	1.75–1.5
	Fair	3.0–2.25	2.25–2.0
	Poor	3.25 or more	2.5 or more
Ankle dorsiflexion	Excellent	26.5 or less	24.25 or less
	Good	29.5–26.75	26.5–24.5
	Average	32.5–29.75	30.25–26.75
	Fair	35.25–32.75	31.75–30.5
	Poor	35.5 or more	32.0 or more

Adapted tests with no normative data

As with the previous adapted tests, only a tape measure is required. There are no normative data for this type of testing so subsequent tests must be compared against baseline test data.

Lumbar flexion

1. The subject stands upright on the floor with the arms by the sides of the body.
2. The tester makes two marks on the body: one in the centre of the back along an imaginary line at the top of the pelvic girdle, and the other 15cm above this.
3. The subject then bends forwards from the trunk as far as possible, keeping the legs straight.
4. Measure the new distance between the points and subtract 15cm from this.

Fig. 5.26   Lumbar flexion

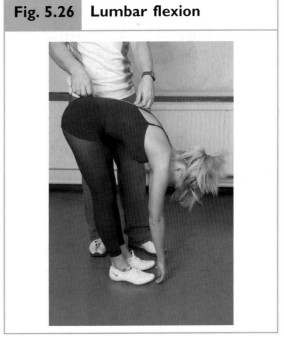

Lumbar extension

1. The subject stands upright on the floor with the arms by the sides of the body.
2. The tester makes two marks on the body: one in the centre of the back along an imaginary line at the top of the pelvic girdle, and the other 15cm above this.
3. The subject then bends backwards from the trunk as far as possible, keeping the legs straight.
4. Measure the new distance between the points and subtract 15cm from this.

Lumbar flexion for the older age group

1. The subject stands upright on the floor with the arms by the sides of the body.
2. The subject then bends forwards from the trunk as far as possible, keeping the legs straight, and reaches towards the floor.
3. Measure the vertical distance from the tips of the fingers to the floor.
4. Repeat the test several times.

| **Fig. 5.28** | **Lumbar flexion for the older age group** |

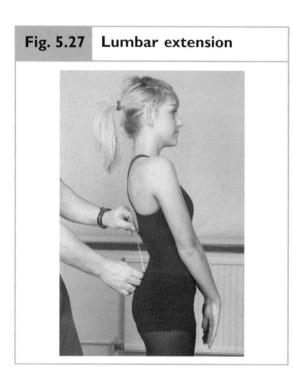

| **Fig. 5.27** | **Lumbar extension** |

Lumbar extension for the older age group

1. The subject stands upright on the floor with the arms by the sides of the body.
2. The subject then bends backwards from the trunk as far as possible, keeping the legs straight.
3. With the palms facing forwards, the subject keeps the arms straight and in a vertical line to the floor.
4. Measure the vertical distance from the tips of the fingers to the floor.
5. Repeat the test several times.

Lateral lumbar flexion

1. The subject stands upright on the floor with the arms by the sides of the body and the palms facing inwards.
2. The feet of the subject should be hip distance apart.
3. The subject then bends sideways from the trunk as far as possible, keeping the legs straight, and reaches towards the floor with a straight arm.
4. Measure the vertical distance from the tips of the fingers to the floor.
5. Repeat the test several times.

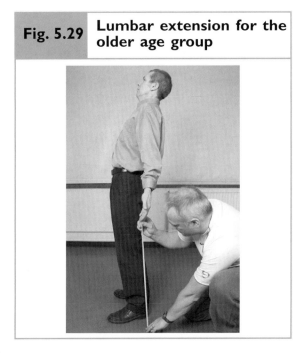

Fig. 5.29 **Lumbar extension for the older age group**

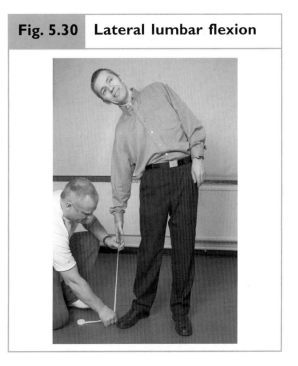

Fig. 5.30 **Lateral lumbar flexion**

Sit-and-reach test

A common indirect flexibility test used frequently in the health and fitness industry is the *sit-and-reach test*. Here an individual sits with straight legs and stretches forwards to record the distance reached with the fingertips. This type of test is common but it is a measure of both hamstring and upper back flexibility depending on the protocol used for the test.

Studies have suggested this test to be an acceptable field-test measure of hamstring flexibility only and not a valid measuring tool for lower back flexibility.

Fig. 5.31 Sit-and-reach test

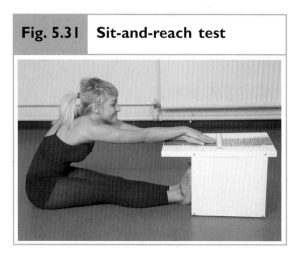

Required resources

A 'sit-and-reach box' or a bench with a ruler.

Testing method

1. Allow the subject to fully warm up and stretch before the start of the test.
2. The subject's legs should be fully extended with the feet (no shoes) flat against the vertical surface of the box.
3. With one hand placed over the other (palms down, arms straight, fingers outstretched), the subject should lean forward as far as possible, sliding their hand along the ruler of the sit-and-reach box.
4. The maximal distance the fingers reach is measured.
5. The subject must keep their hands together and should not lead with one hand.
6. Repeat several times and record the best score.

NEED TO KNOW

The initial investigation by Wells and Dillon in the 1950s was designed to investigate the sit-and-reach test as a test of back and leg flexibility. The equipment used was basic, consisting of a rubber mat, two benches and a platform that included a measuring scale.

Analysis

Typical analysis of flexibility for the sit-and-reach test is by recording the distance achieved and using this either as a baseline measure for subsequent comparison or classifying against a normative-value data set.

There are many arguments relating to the analysis of flexibility measurements. One of the arguments is that joint flexibility should be within a limited range (distance at a certain angle) so as not to compromise joint stability while still allowing a certain degree of flexibility giving the joint mobility. Normative tables, however, make the assumption that the greater the range of flexibility (the higher the score in this case), the better the category for the individual being tested.

Some researchers consider that flexibility beyond a certain limit in a joint may restrict the amount of stability that soft tissue, in particular muscle and its fascia, might be responsible for. This should be taken into account when using normative tables for identifying the classification of flexibility.

Classification

Even though the previous information should be taken into account, tables 5.4a and 5.4b can be used to identify the classification of flexibility for 16-year-olds and adults.

Differences in body size (for instance height and limb length) can all potentially affect sit-and-reach scores, making it difficult to compare subjects to each other. People with long arms and short legs have an advantage over those with short arms and long legs. In most cases, test results will not be affected, except for those with extreme differences. To overcome these issues, a modified sit-and-reach test has been developed by Hoeger and colleagues.

Table 5.4a	Sit-and-reach normative data for 16-year-olds (values in cm)				
Gender	Excellent	Above average	Average	Below average	Poor
Male	>28	24–28	20–23	17–19	<17
Female	>35	32–35	30–31	25–29	<25

Table 5.4b	Sit-and-reach normative data for adults (values in cm)				
Gender	Excellent	Above average	Average	Below average	Poor
Male	>29	26–29	22–25	19–21	<19
Female	>30	27–30	22–26	19–21	<19

Modified sit-and-reach test

Required resources

A 30cm (12-inch) box, metre ruler.

Testing method

1. Allow the subject to fully warm up and stretch before the start of the test.
2. The subject's legs should be fully extended with the feet (no shoes) flat against the vertical surface of the box.
3. The subject should be positioned with their back against a wall, with buttocks, shoulders and head against the wall.
4. Place a metre ruler on top of the box with the zero end pointing towards the subject.
5. The subject should reach forwards with their hands as far as possible with both head and shoulders remaining in contact with the wall (figure 5.32a).
6. Note the distance travelled along the metre stick.
7. The subject should then make three controlled forward movements, leaning forwards as far as possible and holding that position for a two-second period (figure 5.32b).
8. Measure the distance. The difference between this and the distance measured in step 6 is the modified sit-and-reach score. Two trials should be made and the results averaged.

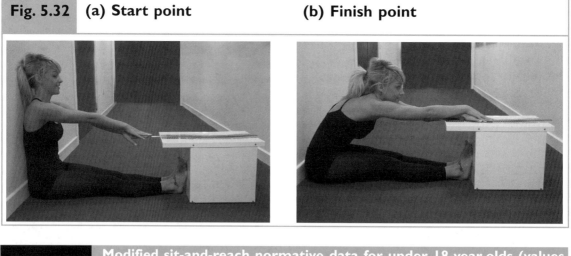

Fig. 5.32 **(a) Start point** **(b) Finish point**

Table 5.5a	Modified sit-and-reach normative data for under 18-year-olds (values in cm)				
Gender	Excellent	Above average	Average	Below average	Poor
Male	>19.6	17.8	14.5	11.8	<8.4
Female	>19.5	17.8	14.5	12.6	<9.4

Table 5.5b	Modified sit-and-reach normative data for adults, 19–35 years old (values in cm)				
Gender	Excellent	Above average	Average	Below average	Poor
Male	>18.9	17.0	14.4	11.6	<7.9
Female	>19.3	16.7	14.8	12.6	<8.1

Further reading

Alter, M. J. (1996) *Science of flexibility*, 2nd edn, Champaign, Illinois: Human Kinetics

Anderson, B. & Anderson, J. (1980) *Stretching*, Bolinas, California: Shelter Publications

Anderson, B. & Burke, E. R. (1991) 'Scientific, medical and practical aspects of stretching'. *Clinics in Sports Medicine*, 10: pp. 63-86

Anderson, O. (2000) 'Does stretching really lower the risk of injury?'. *Sports Injury Bulletin*, 1: pp. 4-9

Bandy, W. D. et al. (1998) 'The effects of a static stretch and dynamic range of motion training on the flexibility of the hamstring muscles'. *Journal of Orthopaedic and Sports Physical Therapy*, 27: pp. 295-300

Bandy, W. D. & Reese, N. B. (2002) *Joint Range of Motion and Muscle Length Testing*, Philadelphia, Pennsylvania: W. B. Saunders

Beaulieu, J. V. et al. (1981) 'Developing a stretching program'. *Physician Sportsmed*, 9: pp. 59-66

Blair, S. N. (1986) 'Rates and risks for running and exercise injuries: Studies in three populations'. *Research Quarterly for Exercise and Sport*, 58: pp. 221-8

Davis, V. G. (1982) 'Flexibility conditioning for running', in D'Ambrosia, R. & Drez, D. (eds.) *Prevention and Treatment of Running Injuries*. Thorofare, New Jersey: Charles B. Slack Inc., pp. 135-45

Dean, C. et al. (1990) 'Viscoelastic properties of muscle-tendon units'. *The American Journal of Sports Medicine*, 18: pp. 300-9

Ekstrand, J. et al (1982) 'Prevention of soccer injuries: Supervision by doctor and physiotherapist'. *American Journal of Sports Medicine*, 10: pp. 75-8

Franks, D. B. (1983) 'Physical warm-up'. In Williams, M. H. (ed.) *Ergogenic Aids in Sport*, Champaign, Illinois: Human Kinetics, pp. 340-75

Gleim, G. W. & McHugh, M. P. (1997) 'Flexibility and its effects on sports injury and performance'. *Sports Medicine*, 24: pp. 289-99

Goldspink, G. (1968) 'Sarcomere length during post-natal growth and mammalian muscle fibres'. *Journal of Cell Science*, 3: pp. 539-48

Halbertsma, J. P. K. et al (1996) 'Sport stretching: Effect on passive muscle stiffness in short hamstrings of healthy subjects'. *Archives of Physical Medicine and Rehabilitation*, 77: pp. 688-92

Heyward, V. H. (2006) *Advanced Fitness Assessment and Exercise Prescription,* 5th edn, Champaign, Illinois: Human Kinetics

Holt, L. E. (1973) *Scientific Stretching for Sport,* Halifax, Nova Scotia: Dalhousie University

Hubley-Kozey, C. L. & Stanish, W. D. (1990) 'Can stretching prevent athletic injuries?' *Journal of Musculoskeletal Medicine,* 7: pp. 21-31

Jacobs, S. J. (1986) 'Injuries to runners: A study of entrants to a 10,000 metre race'. *American Journal of Sports Medicine,* 14: pp. 151-5

Lally, D. (1994) 'New study links stretching with higher injury rates'. *Running Research News,* 10: pp. 5-6

McCullogh, C. (1990) 'Stretching for injury prevention'. *Patient Management,* 14: pp. 79-85

Madding, S. W. (1987) 'Effects of duration of passive stretch on hip abduction range of motion'. *Journal of Orthopaedic Sports Physical Therapy,* 8: pp. 409-416

Magnusson, S. P. et al. (1996) 'Mechanical and Physical responses to stretching with and without pre-isometric contraction in human skeletal muscle'. *Archives of Physical and Medical Rehabilitation,* 77: pp. 373-8

Mann, R. (1982) 'Biomechanics of running', in *Prevention and Treatment of Running Injuries,* Thorofare, New Jersey: Charles B. Slack Inc., pp. 1-13

Moore, M. A. & Hutton, R. S. (1980) 'Electromyographic investigation of muscle stretching techniques'. *Medicine and Science in Sports and Exercise,* 12: pp. 322-9

Noonan, T. J. (1993) 'Thermal effects on skeletal muscle tensile behaviour'. *American Journal of Sports Medicine,* 21: pp. 517-22

Pope, R (1998) 'Effects of ankle dorsiflexion range and pre-exercise calf muscle stretching on injury risk in army recruits'. *Australian Journal of Physiotherapy,* 44: pp. 165-77

Pope, R et al. (2000) 'A randomised trial of pre-exercise stretching for prevention of lower-limb injury'. *Medicine and Science in Sports and Exercise,* 32: pp. 271-7

Richardson, et al. (1999) *Therapeutic Exercises for Spinal Segmental Stabilisation in Low Back Pain,* Oxford, UK: Churchill, Livingstone

Rosenbaum, D. & Hennig, E. M. (1995) 'The influence of stretching and warm up exercises on Achilles tendon reflex activity'. *Journal of Sports Sciences,* 13: pp. 481-90

Saal, J. S. (1987) 'Flexibility training'. *Physical Medicine and Rehabilitation: State of the Art Reviews,* 1: pp. 537-54

Safran, M. R. et al. (1988) 'The role of warm-up in muscular injury prevention'. *American Journal of Sports Medicine,* 16: pp. 123-9

Smith, C. A. (1994) 'The warm-up procedure; to stretch or not to stretch. A brief review'. *Journal of Orthopaedic Sports Physical Therapy,* 19: pp. 12-17

Solveborn, S. A. (1985) *The Book about Stretching,* New York, New York: Japan Publications

Shrier, I. & Gossal, K. (2000) 'Myths and truths of stretching'. *The Physician and Sportsmedicine,* 28: pp. 57-63

Stark, S. D. (1997) *Stretching techniques in the stark reality of stretching*, Richmond, British Colombia: Stark Reality Publishing, pp. 73-80

Taylor, D. C. et al (1990) 'Viscoelastic properties of muscle-tendon units'. *The American Journal of Sports Medicine*, 18: pp. 300-9

Thomas, J. R. & Nelson, J. K. (1996) *Research Methods in Physical Activity,* 3rd edn, Champaign, Illinois: Human Kinetics

Van Mechelen, W. (1993) 'Prevention of running injuries by warm-up, cool-down, and stretching exercises'. *The American Journal of Sports Medicine*, 22: pp. 711-19

Wells, K. F. & Dillon, E. K. (1952) 'The sit and reach – a test of back and leg flexibility'. *Research Quarterly*, 23: pp. 115-18

Wolpaw, J. R. & Carp, J. S. (1990) 'Memory traces in spinal cord'. *Trends in Neuroscience*, 13: pp. 137-42

Worrell, T. W. (1994) 'Factors associated with hamstrings injuries: An approach to treatment and preventative measures'. *Sports Medicine*, 17: pp. 338-45

Yamaguchi, T., Ishil K., Yamanaka, M. & Yasuda, K. (2007) 'Acute effects of dynamic stretching exercise on power output during concentric dynamic constant external resistance leg extension'. *Journal of Strength and Conditioning Research*, 21(4): pp. 1238-44

Young, W. B. & Behm, D. G. (2003) 'Effects of running, static stretching and practice jumps on explosive force production and jumping performance'. *Journal of Sports Medicine and Physical Fitness*, 43: pp. 21-7

Young, W., Clothier, P., Otago, L., Bruce, L. & Liddell, D. (2004) 'Acute effects of static stretching on hip flexor and quadriceps flexibility, range of motion and foot speed in kicking a football'. *Journal of Science and Medicine in Sport*, 7: pp. 3-31

Yuktasir, B. Kaya, F. (2009) 'Investigation into the long-term effects of static and PNF stretching exercises on range of motion and jump performance'. *Journal of Bodywork and Movement Therapies*, 13: pp. 11–21

Zakas, A. (2004) 'The effect of stretching duration on the lower-extremity flexibility of adolescent soccer players'. *Journal of Bodywork and Movement Therapies*, 9: pp. 220-5

Zakas, A., Balaska, P., Grammatikopoulou, M. G., Zakas, N. & Vergon, A. (2005) 'Acute effects of stretching duration on the range of motion of elderly women'. *Journal of Bodywork and Movement Therapies*, 9: pp. 270-6

Zakas, A., Dognis, G., Papakonstandinon, V., Sentelidis, T. & Vamvakondis, E., (2006) 'Acute effects of static stretching duration on isokinetic peak torque production of soccer players'. *Journal of Bodywork and Movement Therapies*, 10: pp. 89-95

MUSCULAR STRENGTH AND ENDURANCE TESTING

6

OBJECTIVES

After completing this chapter you should be able to:

1 Explain the terms 'strength', 'force', 'isometric', 'eccentric', 'concentric', 'isokinetic' and 'muscular endurance'.

2 Discuss the importance of muscular strength for particular populations such as older people.

3 List and discuss each of the factors that determine muscular strength and endurance.

4 Understand the advantages and disadvantages of strength testing using free weights versus machine weights.

5 Explain the use of different protocols and the effectiveness of sub-maximal testing for determining 1RM.

6 Recognise how strength is affected by gender, age, velocity of movement, and joint angle.

7 List and describe a range of tests that are commonly used for assessing muscular strength.

8 List and describe a range of tests that are commonly used for assessing muscular endurance.

Muscular strength

Measurement of muscular strength is useful from both a health and an exercise performance perspective; strength training has an important role in both young and elderly populations.

Regular exercise can generally be considered to be more important in elderly groups than in any others. As a consequence of ageing, there is a loss of strength due to disuse and atrophy (muscle shrinkage), which can often result in a decreased ability to function by oneself and an increased reliance on others. Even simple tasks like getting out of a chair or onto a bus require a minimum level of muscular strength.

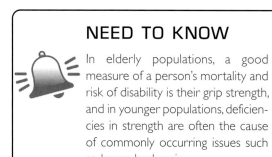

NEED TO KNOW

In elderly populations, a good measure of a person's mortality and risk of disability is their grip strength, and in younger populations, deficiencies in strength are often the cause of commonly occurring issues such as lower back pain.

Strength testing is useful in showing the imbalances between limbs (dominant and non-dominant limbs) and between muscle groups (hamstring to quadriceps ratio, for example), which can lead to an increase in injury risk. In addition, when rehabilitating from injury, measurements of strength can provide a guide to how well the individual is recovering and can therefore help in estimating when they might reach full fitness. However, one of the main reasons for strength testing is to provide feedback for development and evaluation of resistance training programmes (Coulson and Archer 2008).

As it has been shown that gains in strength as a result of resistance training can vary from 2 per cent in elite athletes to 40 per cent in untrained individuals (ACSM 2002), it is important (particularly in elite groups) that testing is carried out on a regular basis and that the accuracy of the associated measurements used is high.

Definitions

It is useful to be aware of, and understand, some of the terminology commonly, and often incorrectly, used in relation to muscular strength.

Many definitions of strength have been proposed over the years. As far back as 1935, it was defined by Arthur Steindler as *'the maximal display of contractile power'* and in 1966 Henry Harrison Clarke tried to refine the statement by removing the concept of power and stated that *'muscular strength is the tension that muscles can apply in a single maximum contraction'*.

The view that strength has many components (such as static, dynamic and explosive) has been debated for many years, with opponents stating that these components are not independent.

Strength has also been defined as *'the ability of the neuromuscular system to produce force in a single contraction at a specific velocity'*. Strength is also frequently referred to as maximum force or torque. Forces are often perceived as pushes or pulls and can be defined as the ability to accelerate, decelerate, stop or change the direction of an object. Force is calculated as mass multiplied by acceleration (i.e. $F = ma$).

The units of force are known as Newtons (N) or pounds (lbs) and torque is the product of force multiplied by moment arm length (the distance from the pivot to the force causing the torque) and is measured in Newton metres (Nm). When performing strength testing with equipment such as a dynamometer, it is actually torque (turning force) that is being measured (figure 6.1).

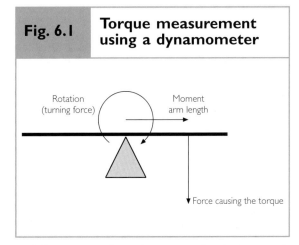

Fig. 6.1 Torque measurement using a dynamometer

Rotation (turning force)

Moment arm length

Force causing the torque

When a muscle is shortening (under tension) during a movement such as a biceps-curl exercise (figure 6.2a), the contraction is termed *concentric*. When the weight is lowered in a controlled manner under tension and the muscles are lengthening, it is known as an *eccentric* muscle action (figure 6.2b). When the muscle is under tension but there is no movement, this is defined as an *isometric* muscle action (figure 6.2c).

The term *isotonic* (constant tension) is used extensively to describe muscle activity where the resistance is constant, such as in moving or lifting free weights. This definition is actually incorrect as the force during nearly all movements is never constant; it is affected by factors such as the angle of the joint or movement velocity.

Some researchers prefer to use the term *isoinertial* or *dynamic constant external resistance* as it more accurately describes what occurs in the muscle when moving constant masses such as free weights (for a more detailed explanation please refer to the references at the end of the chapter).

When a limb moves at a constant speed regardless of the resistance applied to it, this is termed an *isokinetic* movement. Specialised

| Fig. 6.2 | **Concentric (a), eccentric (b) and isometric (c) phases of a bicep curl** |

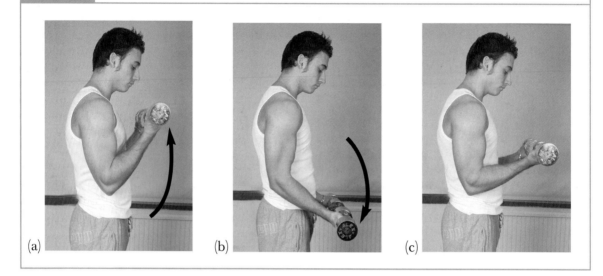

(a)   (b)   (c)

equipment can be used to measure force at a constant speed. This type of equipment is usually called an isokinetic dynamometer.

Factors determining muscle strength

In testing for muscle strength and endurance, it is useful to understand the factors that could affect or determine the strength and endurance of an individual.

Although genetics plays an important role in the potential development of strength and endurance, training can also contribute to development to some extent. The force that can be developed by an individual during muscle shortening or lengthening is dependent on many physiological and biomechanical factors, some of which can be affected by training. These factors include:

- Muscle cross-sectional area
- Contraction velocity
- Muscle length
- Fibre arrangement
- Tendon insertion
- Nervous system recruitment
- Fibre type

Muscle cross-sectional area

It is generally considered that the main factor in determining the strength of a muscle or muscle group is its cross-sectional area (CSA). It is believed that the greater the cross-sectional area of the muscle, the greater the capability for that muscle to generate force.

One of the known effects of strength (resistance) training is muscular hypertrophy (increase in muscle mass), and varying the exercises, intensity and volume can affect the muscle mass gains. The use of very heavy weights (near maximal) is typically associated with gains in strength with moderate hypertrophy, whereas the use of moderately heavy weights (and high volume of training) as used by bodybuilders is more typically associated with gains in muscle mass (Coulson and Archer 2008). It has been demonstrated on many occasions that the gains in strength, in subjects who are considered untrained, as a result of 3–5 months of resistance training, are mainly associated with gains in cross-sectional area of the muscle.

Contraction velocity

The speed of the muscle contraction (and hence the movement) can affect the forces that can be developed (figure 6.3) within the muscle. In simple terms, during concentric muscle contraction, the faster the muscular contraction the less force is produced. It is generally thought that this is due to a lower number of cross-bridge connections within the muscle being involved at higher velocities. (The relationship between force and velocity is further explained in chapter 8.)

With strength testing, most tests such as the one repetition maximum (1RM) test are performed at low velocities during concentric exercises.

Muscle length

It has been demonstrated (not just in research associated with muscle testing but in calculations used in engineering modelling as well) that the joint angle can have a large effect on the ability of the muscle to generate force.

When performing biceps curls (elbow flexion – see figure 6.2) for example, the torque that can be developed is at its highest between the angles of 70 and 120°.

At 0°, when the bar is at the lowest position, with the arms fully extended, it is difficult to lift the resistance because the joint angle is not favourable (no force angle is available). Individuals will often 'cheat' at this point by first bending their trunk forward to create momentum and a more favourable joint angle in order to lift the resistance. This often happens when people try to lift a weight that is too heavy for them to lift with correct form. This is due to the number of cross-bridge heads in alignment with binding sites being greatest at around the resting length of muscles.

Fibre arrangement

In relation to the alignment of muscle fibres, some muscles have fibres that lie in parallel to the long axis of the muscle, and some muscles have fibres that lie at an oblique angle (these are called *pennate* muscles). Pennate muscles have a greater ability to generate force in relation to non-pennate muscles of the same cross-sectional area. The angle of pennation within individual muscles is determined genetically; this helps to explain why some people are able to generate more force than others using the same muscle group.

Tendon insertion

Tendons (which attach muscle to bone) primarily comprise a substance called *collagen*, which

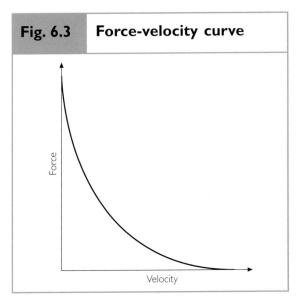

| Fig. 6.3 | **Force-velocity curve** |

Force

Velocity

is tightly packed in parallel bundles. Tendons are slightly elastic and connect to either bone or cartilage. The force of muscle contraction is transmitted through muscle fibres, via the tendons to the bone. Mechanical forces as a result of strength training can stimulate growth and strength of the tendon tissue, depending on the intensity and frequency of the exercises being carried out. There are three sites at which the tendon tissue can increase strength:

1. The junction between the tendon and the bone surface
2. Within the body of the tendon
3. Within the connective tissue fascia network of the muscle

The exact adaptive mechanism within tendon tissue that occurs as a result of regular strength training is complex. However, it is generally known that the adaptation that does occur increases the ability of the tendon to withstand greater tension.

Nervous system recruitment

Neural factors are considered to be strong determinants of strength. The majority of strength gains in the first eight weeks of resistance training are achieved by increased activation of the nervous system as it undergoes what could be described as a learning process. One of the neural factors thought to assist in the development of strength is the improvement of recruitment patterns during muscular contraction. It has been suggested that resistance training is responsible for a more precise and efficient motor-unit recruitment.

Fibre type

As previously discussed, muscle fibre-type distribution is genetically determined. However, there is a certain amount of adaptation of the fibres that can be achieved as a result of training.

It has often been demonstrated that athletes who regularly train for events such as weightlifting or sprinting have a larger proportion of type II (fast-twitch) muscle fibres than those athletes involved in endurance events, whereas those athletes who train regularly for endurance events have a larger proportion of type I (slow-twitch) fibres compared to those in strength or sprint events.

Strength-testing protocol

Muscular strength is a component of fitness (see chapter 2) that is considered to be a requirement in the performance of many sports or athletic events. However, due to the complex nature of strength training and subsequent adaptation there are many issues that should be addressed by the coach and athlete when developing a strength-testing protocol. Some of the key issues often include the following:

- How reliable is the testing procedure?
- What is the relationship between the test results and performance?
- Is the test measurement valid for the individual and/or the activity?
- Is the test sensitive enough to detect the effects of training or rehabilitation?
- Does the test distinguish between groups and within groups?
- Are there any normative values for comparison?
- Is the subject capable of performing the test?

When selecting strength tests one of the main questions asked should be '*what and who is being tested?*' Testing methods can vary depending on what is being measured and the type of athlete being tested.

Although there is no single isolated test that can be used to evaluate all types of strength, there are two types of strength testing that can be broadly categorised as *isometric* and *isokinetic*.

Isometric testing

This method simply tests strength at a particular angle of a joint.

As explained earlier in this chapter, muscular force development is affected by movement velocity (contraction speed of the muscle). Isometric testing essentially overcomes this problem since, by definition, the speed of an isometric muscle contraction is zero ($0°s^{-1}$), as the muscle is held in a static position.

Isometric strength testing has been used for the last 60 years because it is easy to standardise, needs little technique on the part of the subject, is relatively safe and simple to perform, and is inexpensive compared to other strength tests.

Depending on the type of isometric testing equipment used, the test can determine parameters such as maximal force, maximal torque, and rate of force development (RFD). Rate of force development is a useful measure, as it determines the muscular force that can be generated in the early phases of muscle contraction (approximately 0–200ms), and increases rapidly as a result of undertaking a regular period of heavy resistance training. Rate of force development can be measured as the time to reach a specific force, time to reach a relative force (for example 50 per cent of maximum force), or by the slope of the force-time curve as produced in figure 6.4.

One of the limitations of isometric testing is that there is often a poor relationship between the measures obtained involving no movement and dynamic performance measures such as 1RM, sprint speed, vertical jump or throwing and punching speed.

The available research evidence would tend

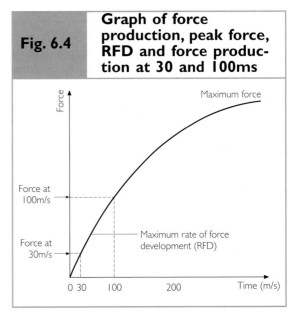

Fig. 6.4 Graph of force production, peak force, RFD and force production at 30 and 100ms

to indicate that dynamic measures of muscular function are more valid than isometric measures when assessing functional capacity during dynamic activities. One reason for this may be that there is no involvement of the stretch-shortening cycle (SSC) in isometric testing. This is unfortunate as the stretch-shortening cycle and the elastic nature of tissue are integral to nearly all movements such as a vertical jump and sprinting. Nonetheless, isometric testing is still frequently performed in both clinical and sporting environments.

Over the last 50 years isometric strength of the back and hip has been assessed at multiple joints through the use of *tensiometers*, which measure strain on a cable produced by muscular action (see figure 6.5). More recently, the use of strain gauges and force transducers has been developed to measure the forces.

Performing actions with the body in different positions leads to an assessment of either back or hip strength. The advantages of these techniques are that the equipment is relatively inexpensive, portable, and easy and safe to operate.

Researchers at Liverpool John Moores

University have found that the technique of portable dynamometry is valid in the measurement of back and hip strength, provided that the measurement protocol is standardised. One of the limitations of these tests, however, is that incorrect technique can produce spurious values, and it does not give information about bi-lateral imbalances (differences between dominant and non-dominant sides of the body).

More recently, several researchers have developed new techniques for assessing isometric strength through the use of laboratory-type equipment known as a *force plate*. Force plates look like a metal box (about 1m^2 in size) which is placed in the ground, flush with the surface, and will measure any force (and direction of that force) that is directed upon it.

For isometric strength testing, the force plate can measure the ground reaction force (the amount and direction of the force) resulting from the subject pushing on a bar that has been fixed in place.

These methods have been developed and used for assessing isometric strength when performing bench press, back squat, shoulder press, dead-lift, upright row, arm curl and a range of other exercises. These multi-joint testing methods are considered to be reasonably reliable and more representative of athletic performance than testing with leg or back tensiometers.

In relation to commonly performed isometric strength testing, *grip strength* is one of the most frequently chosen methods used by coaches and instructors. It does, however, have many limitations, as it is really only a measure of the strength of the forearm muscles and not overall muscle strength. Despite this, it is commonly used in team sports such as rugby and soccer because it is inexpensive, easy to operate and quick to administer even with a large group of subjects. It could also be argued that the only time a soccer player would be using their grip strength is in holding on to an opponent's shirt or body, which is not officially permitted.

Fig. 6.5	A typical tensiometer in use

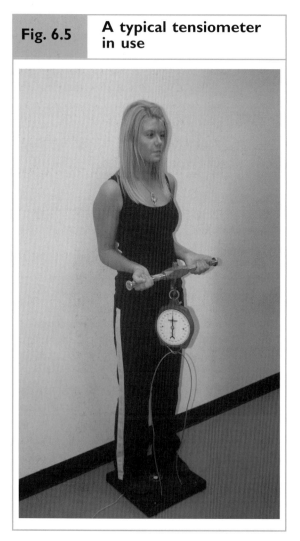

Tensiometer strength tests

Tensiometers can be used to test isometric strength of various body parts such as the legs or back.

Required resources

Tensiometer, tape measure.

Assessment of leg strength

1. Instruct the subject to undertake a warm-up and minimal stretching before testing.
2. Subjects should wear appropriate footwear such as training shoes.
3. They should stand flat on the footplate (15cm from the wall) with scapulae and buttocks positioned flat against the wall.
4. The body should slide down the wall until the legs are flexed to 135° (assessed by goniometry) and subjects should have the elbows fully extended.
5. The bar should be placed in the subject's hands (cable length adjusted for height).
6. Subjects should be instructed to extend the legs with maximal effort, pulling the bar simultaneously.
7. Record the maximum (kg) of three attempts.

Assessment of back strength

1. As for testing leg strength, subjects should be instructed to warm up, stretch minimally and wear appropriate footwear.
2. They should stand flat on the footplate (15cm from the wall) with legs kept straight and the back flexed at the hip.
3. Elbows should be fully extended and back flexion continued until the tips of the index fingers meet the patellae.
4. The bar should be placed in the subject's hands (cable length adjusted for height). Reverse grip should be used to minimise use of shoulder muscles during the movement.
5. Subjects should be instructed to keep the head up and extend the back with maximal effort, maintaining a strong grip.
6. Record the maximum (kg) of three attempts.

Fig. 6.6	**(a) Leg tensiometer test**	**(b) Back tensiometer test**

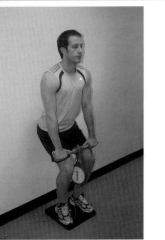 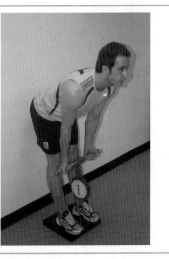

Grip strength test

Required resources

Handgrip dynamometer.

Testing method

1. Ensure the dynamometer is set to zero.
2. Adjust the hand grip to suit the subject. The handle should rest on the middle phalanges and the base on the first metacarpal.
3. Raise the dynamometer above the head with palms facing inwards.
4. Take a deep breath and squeeze the handle as hard as possible while lowering the arm over a three-second period, elbows fully extended.
5. Record the maximum reading (kg) from three attempts, alternating between the dominant and non-dominant hand.

Analysis

Analysis can be done by comparing the results with those of previous tests. It is expected that, with appropriate training between tests, this would indicate an improvement in the subject's grip strength. A handgrip strength of 150N (approximately 15kg), equivalent to 20 per cent of bodyweight for a 75kg individual, is a suggested threshold for occupational tasks requiring a firm grip. For a 25-year-old male, a grip strength of 30kg is very poor, but the same measurement of 30kg for a 75-year-old male is average to good.

Classification

See table 6.1.

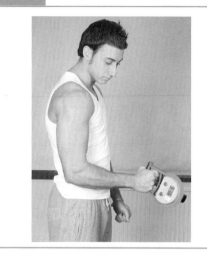

Fig. 6.7 **Grip strength test using a dynamometer**

NEED TO KNOW

Researchers in the USA found that grip strength measured in over 6,000 45–68-year-old males was a good predictor of disability and functional limitations 25 years later (Rantanen et al. 1999). This included the ability to rise from a chair or walk faster than 1.4 km/h indicating that good muscle strength in midlife can prevent or delay the onset of old age disability. Grip strength in the elderly is actually a better predictor of frailty than chronological age (Syddall et al. 2003).

Table 6.1	Normative values for grip strength (kg)				
Gender	Excellent	Good	Average	Fair	Poor
Male	>56	51–56	45–50	39–44	<39
Female	>36	31–36	25–30	19–24	<19

Isokinetic testing

One measurement of strength commonly performed in laboratories and rehabilitation centres is *maximal voluntary contraction* (MVC). This type of strength testing is frequently performed using machines known as *isokinetic dynamometers.*

When testing strength using typical resistance machines or free weights, the velocities change between repetitions and throughout the movement. Isokinetic dynamometry was first developed in the late 1960s to overcome such limitations by using hydraulic or electromechanical systems to maintain constant angular velocity.

Most dynamometry systems can test the strength of the core and all major upper- and lower-body muscles (measurement of isometric, concentric and eccentric strength can all be performed using this type of equipment). As these machines are relatively expensive, their use is mainly confined to clinical environments such as hospitals/rehabilitation centres, research institutes, universities, and teams in highly paid professional sports such as soccer, rugby and American football.

The values obtained are very reproducible (5 per cent day-to-day variability), but comparisons between different dynamometers are problematic. Different models and manufacturers can result in differences of 5–10 per cent in torque measured using different dynamometers.

When performing isokinetic assessments of strength, the following settings should be considered:

- Angular velocity and order
- Number of repetitions
- Rest intervals
- Range of motion
- Contraction modes
- Positioning and stabilisation

The *angular velocity* can be controlled between $0°s^{-1}$ and $500°s^{-1}$ depending on the system. Units used are either $°s^{-1}$ or radians per second ($rad.s^{-1}$); $1\ rad.s^{-1} = 57.3°s^{-1}$.

As mentioned previously, force decreases with increasing velocity (see figure 6.3) and the accuracy of velocities is typically around $1°s^{-1}$. Training at a specific velocity results in greatest improvements around that velocity and thus training at a range of velocities of between $180°$ and $240°s^{-1}$ would seem to be the best recommendation.

In terms of velocity selection, the nature of the movement in the specific sport should be considered. When performing isokinetic tests, the typical order is from slowest to fastest and the following velocities are commonly used: $60°s^{-1}$, $90°s^{-1}$, $120°s^{-1}$, $180°s^{-1}$, $240°s^{-1}$ and $360°s^{-1}$. (A common procedure is to test at $60°s^{-1}$, $240°s^{-1}$ and then $360°s^{-1}$). Subjects are more comfortable working at lower velocities and may need some extra practice when performing at higher velocities.

The *number of repetitions* used should be at least 3–5, as the greatest values are typically reached by repetition two or three (see figure 6.8). For tests of muscular endurance, between 30 and 50 repetitions are typically used. The duration of time between sets can be set prior to testing and a *rest interval* of at least 40 to 90 seconds should be allowed to minimise the effects of fatigue. The *range of motion* affects many of the measurements obtained (for example average torque). Torque varies throughout the ROM and ROM is normally set on a dynamometer as a safety limit (i.e. a limit beyond which subject safety may be compromised).

In comparing results obtained to those from published literature, the ROM used should be identified. When performing repeated tests on the same individual, the ROM should be standardised and set similarly each time.

The *contraction modes* can be set on most

dynamometers for concentric or eccentric muscle actions; a typical test setting is knee extension followed by flexion, which can be used for setting agonist/antagonist ratios.

Positioning and stabilisation of the joints about which torque is being assessed is vital from both a safety and a measurement reliability perspective. Significant forces may be developed when large muscle masses are being recruited and, if the measurements are not being performed along the correctly identified axis, injury can occur.

The axis of rotation of the dynamometer lever should be in line with the centre of rotation of the joint being assessed. This is easier with some joints; for example the knee joint is easier to assess than other joints such as the shoulder.

The stabilisation of the joint ensures that movement around only the joint of interest is assessed; therefore straps should be securely positioned, but should not cause pain.

Gripping dynamometer handles (if present) when performing a typical knee extension/ flexion has been found to result in increased torque production, and hence whether gripping is permitted or not must be kept consistent for each subject.

Many subjects are not familiar with being tested on an isokinetic dynamometer and so brief, clear instructions should be provided, otherwise they may be worried about injuring themselves and not give maximal effort. They should also be given the opportunity to perform some sub-maximal repetitions, especially before testing at greater velocities.

Finally, encouragement should be standardised for each test and consist of clear, concise instructions such as 'push or pull as hard and as fast as possible'.

There are many advantages of isokinetic testing. For instance, it is reliable and reproducible, and can provide information about both dominant and non-dominant limbs, identifying

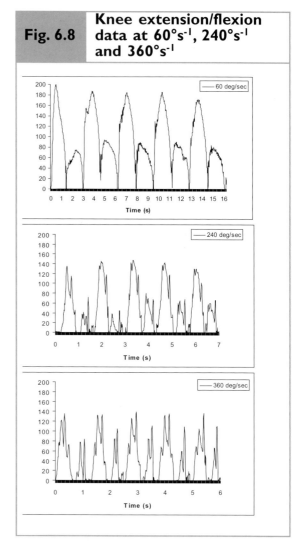

Fig. 6.8 Knee extension/flexion data at 60°s⁻¹, 240°s⁻¹ and 360°s⁻¹

strength imbalances missed by other methods of strength assessment. This type of testing can also isolate joint and muscle groups and can be used safely even if injury is present.

The main disadvantage of isokinetic testing is the need for expensive equipment and the space required to accommodate that equipment. It also takes a relatively long period of time for each subject to be measured and hence would not be suitable in scenarios such as testing an entire team during a single session.

Another potential limitation is that the contraction speeds typically used in isokinetic testing are substantially lower than those speeds obtained during sporting activities that incorporate sprinting-type movements or when playing racquet sports.

Analysis

Figure 6.8 shows the data obtained from testing a 45-year-old man performing a dominant-knee extension/flexion test at $60°s^{-1}$, $240°s^{-1}$ and $360°s^{-1}$. Note the decrease in torque production with increasing velocity and the greater torques obtained during extension compared to flexion. This data could be used to estimate hamstring to quadriceps strength ratio (H:Q ratio). For this subject, his H:Q ratio is 0.46, 0.49 and 0.89 at increasing velocities.

Previously it was thought that this ratio could provide information about injury risks and aptitudes for particular sports such as sprinting, but this is no longer the case. This ratio is affected by velocity, so a simple ratio of 0.6 cannot be selected as the 'correct' ratio between the agonist and antagonist muscles and, in athletes, typically varies between 0.55 and 0.65 at a velocity of $60°s^{-1}$.

An isokinetic dynamometer provides a great deal of data, and common parameters measured include those illustrated in figure 6.8. Peak torque, recorded in Newton-metres (Nm), is one of the most commonly used measures and can be described as the greatest torque achieved during the movement. Dividing this value by the subject's body mass gives the relative peak torque in $Nm.kg^{-1}$. Average peak torque is the average of all the peak torques for each repetition. Average torque is the average torque for the entire torque curve (Nm). Peak power in Watts (W) can also be obtained by multiplying the peak torque by the angular velocity in radians per second.

Classification

Example: Data from 122 outfield professional soccer players indicate a peak torque of 224Nm (relative $2.90Nm.kg^{-1}$) during knee extension, and a peak torque of 165Nm during knee flexion, resulting in a hamstrings/quadriceps strength ratio of 0.74 at $120°s^{-1}$.

Differences in strength of more than 10–15 per cent between limbs can indicate a potential imbalance but care must be taken as some sports (for example tennis) automatically lead to greater development of the dominant arm.

Torque measurements can be used to determine the degree of recovery from injury. Very often the *contra-lateral* (opposite) limb is used to compare the injured limb, and players are often deemed fit to 'return to play' when the returned strength of the injured limb is close to that of the non-injured one. When doing this, the testers and coaches should be aware that the non-injured limb is also likely to decrease in strength due to reduced use and that there are often differences in strength between dominant and non-dominant limbs. Having a series of strength measurements made on both limbs prior to the injury occurring would provide much more useful information in terms of rehabilitation from injury.

Isoinertial testing

Some of the benefits and limitations of isometric and isokinetic testing have already been outlined and, in most practical situations, the most common methods for assessing strength use resistance (see the definition of isoinertial strength testing on page 121). The resistance used can be in the form of external weights such as bars and dumbbells, or can be the individual's body mass as is typically the case in tests of muscular endurance (for example the push-up test).

Strength training is most commonly performed using free weights and machines, and it would make sense to use the same methods to *assess* strength, as subjects would be familiar and comfortable with the techniques.

The movements involved in strength testing using free weights are more similar to those performed in sporting activities, as they require balance and stability. Free weights are relatively inexpensive, widely available and allow complex total body, multiple-joint movements such as power cleans, which would not be possible with machine weights.

One of the potential limitations of the use of free weights is the greater motor control required, increasing the risk of injury compared to machine weights (mainly for those subjects with little experience of training with free weights). This may indicate that strength testing with free weights would be more suitable for healthy athletes, and machine weights for the frail, elderly, injured or those with specific health problems such as arthritis. Another option is to use machine weights to assess strength until sufficient strength and coordination is achieved by the subject before using free-weight testing methods.

In most cases (e.g. bench press) it is maximal concentric strength that is measured. Maximal strength is usually determined from tests involving a low number of repetitions, typically 1–3 repetition maximum (1–3RM). 1RM is more representative of maximal effort, but 2–3RM testing is sometimes preferred as it is more reliable and has a decreased injury risk.

Familiarisation with test procedures is very important for all testing, but especially for strength testing using free weights. The complex nature of some exercises such as Olympic-style lifts requires an extensive period of familiarisation. Increases in strength from strength training may otherwise be overestimated, as they will include the increase in strength simply due to familiarisation with the procedures. This has

often been estimated to range from 10 to 20 per cent in previously untrained individuals.

The reproducibility of 1RM testing in strength-trained athletes is very high, with correlations of between 0.9 and 0.99. It should be noted that there is some evidence to show that when assessing strength using 1RM, it may require more practice sessions to achieve reliable measures for the elderly compared to younger subjects.

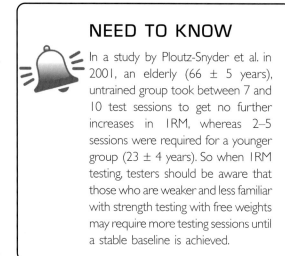

NEED TO KNOW

In a study by Ploutz-Snyder et al. in 2001, an elderly (66 ± 5 years), untrained group took between 7 and 10 test sessions to get no further increases in 1RM, whereas 2–5 sessions were required for a younger group (23 ± 4 years). So when 1RM testing, testers should be aware that those who are weaker and less familiar with strength testing with free weights may require more testing sessions until a stable baseline is achieved.

The risk of injury in performing 1RM is present but may be overestimated, as many studies involving the young and elderly have shown limited injury risk. However, safety must be considered when performing strength testing with free weights or machines. Safety considerations should include the following:

- Weight-lifting equipment such as collars or bars must be checked periodically to see that they have not been damaged.
- The lifting racks used (e.g. squat racks) must be capable of supporting the weights that will be applied.
- The use of spotters increases the safety of testing. The spotter should be trained and

assist in the execution of the lift, and motivate the subject to reach maximal values.

- Spotters must be aware of, and promote, proper technique and must be sufficiently strong to be able to hold heavy weights.
- Spotters must be positioned close to the lifter but not so close as to interfere with the lift.
- If more than one spotter is required, they should have good communication between themselves or otherwise the risk of injury may be increased.

When the subject performs strength tests with free weights it is important that the protocol is standardised. Changes such as grip, arm or foot position can all affect the outcome of the 1RM that is achieved. Starting position is also important, as a greater 1RM will be achieved in an exercise such as the bench press if the subject lowers the bar and then pushes upwards (eccentric then concentric), compared to pushing the bar from chest level (concentric only). This is due to the added harnessing of energy from the stretch-shortening cycle (Coulson and Archer 2008). For some exercises (e.g. squat), varying the body position at the 'depth' of the lift can also affect the values obtained. If the thighs are not lowered to a parallel position in a squat test, the movement will be more like a half-squat and the 1RM values obtained will be inflated (see figures 6.9a and 6.9b).

Note: There is a risk of fatigue if too many repetitions are performed before 1RM is achieved. This can be minimised by providing sufficient rest between repetitions (usually two minutes).

Sub-maximal predictions of 1RM

Many equations have been developed over the years in order to predict 1RM from the number of repetitions performed using lighter weights (known as multiple RMs). This seeks to cater for people for whom maximum weight capacity would not be appropriate. It is important, however, that the set performed during testing is always performed to failure (often termed *volitional failure*). In other words, a 10RM value should mean that no more than 10 repetitions are possible by the subject being tested with the particular weight being used, and they should acknowledge failure on the 11th repetition.

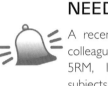

NEED TO KNOW

A recent study by Reynolds and colleagues (2006) determined 1RM, 5RM, 10RM and 20RM in 70 subjects. They found that the best predictions of 1RM were obtained from 5RM testing, and the poorest from 20RM tests. It is recommended not to use more than 10 repetitions when predicting 1RM.

There are many different equations that can be used to predict 1RM from multiple-RM values, but it should be noted that each of the equations gives a different result from the same multiple-RM values that have been measured.

Most research shows that there is a good correlation in predicting 1RM from 6–10RM values (correlation value of r from 0.83 to 0.95). Some investigators, however, have found that the most commonly used equations for predicting 1RM often differ between resistance-trained and untrained subjects. They have further suggested that differences can be found for certain exercises such as knee extensions, leg curls and sit-ups, but cannot be found for others such as bench press and leg press. Some of the more common 1RM prediction equations are those suggested by Brzycki, Lander and Mayhew.

| Fig. 6.9 | (a) A full-squat | (b) A half-squat |

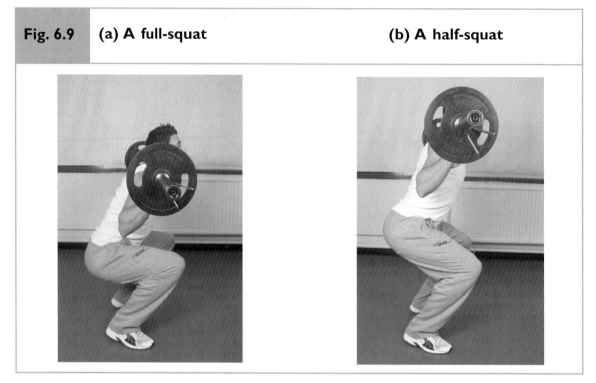

The Brzycki equation (1993)

$$\% \; 1RM = 102.78 - 2.78(\text{repetitions})$$

Example: For 10 repetitions,
$$\% \; 1RM = 102.78 - 2.78(10)$$
Therefore $\% \; 1RM = 75\%$

According to the Brzycki equation, the value of 10RM is equal (or predicted to be equal) to 75.0 per cent of the 1RM value. So, for example, if a subject was tested and measured to have a 10RM of 60 kg, then it follows that 60kg would be 75 per cent of that subject's potential 1RM value. Therefore, for that particular subject, predicted 1RM would be $60/0.75 = 80.0$ kg. Table 6.2 shows predicted percentage of 1RM compared to multiple RM values.

Other sub-maximal 1RM prediction equations have also been suggested by different researchers. Another equation commonly used by strength coaches and instructors to predict 1RM values from multiple efforts for their athletes is the equation proposed by Lander in 1985. This simple-to-use equation is as follows:

$$\% \; 1RM = 101.3 - 2.67123(\text{repetitions})$$

Using the same data as in the Brzycki calculation example earlier where a 10RM of a subject was calculated to be 60kg and hence resulting in a 1RM value of 80kg, for the Lander equation this would result in a 1RM predicted value of 80.4kg. This result differs to the Brzycki result by 0.4kg. This may not seem much but can be the difference between winning and losing in competition. The Lander equation tends to overestimate calculations of 1RM by between 1.5 and 2.5kg.

Table 6.2	Prediction value of %1RM derived from the maximum number of repetitions (RMs) performed
Maximum reps (RM)	% 1RM
1	100
2	95
3	93
4	90
5	87
6	85
7	83
8	80
9	77
10	75
12	67
15	65

1RM squat

Remember that this is a maximal test that is normally only appropriate for individuals with resistance training experience.

Required resources

Relevant weightlifting equipment (Smith machine if available), spotter.

Testing method

1. Subjects warm up. Aim for four lifts and allow rest periods of 3–5 minutes.
2. Subject should begin in an upright position with feet at shoulder width.
3. The subject should descend to a knee angle of 90° of flexion (figure 6.10) and then return to starting point.
4. Weight is progressively increased by 2.5–10kg until lift cannot be performed.
5. Greatest weight successfully completed is the 1RM and this can be divided by the subject's body mass to provide relative 1RM.

Fig. 6.10 **1RM squat test**

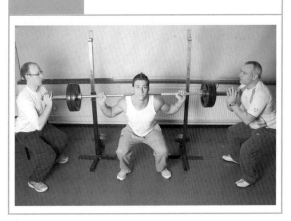

1RM bench press

Required resources

Barbell, weights and bench, spotter.

Testing method

1. Subjects warm up. Aim for four lifts and allow rest periods of 3–5 minutes.
2. Subject lies supine on bench with knees flexed at 90° and feet resting on the bench (can reduce subject's tendency to cheat by using rocking motion of the body to lift the weight).
3. Elbows should be flexed at 90° and arms abducted to 90°.
4. The subject should push the bar until the elbows are fully extended (figure 6.11) and then return to starting point.
5. Weight is progressively increased by 2.5–5kg until lift cannot be performed.
6. Greatest weight successfully completed is the 1RM and this can be divided by the subject's body mass to provide relative 1RM (table 6.4).

Classification

Once the values of the 1RM squat and bench press have been established, tables 6.3 and 6.4 can be used to classify subjects according to gender and age for both squat and bench press.

Many individuals would question the effectiveness of 1RM measures of strength, due to the muscle contractions being less dynamic and in different movement patterns than those typically observed in sporting situations. Although these differences do exist, there is reasonable evidence of links between 1RM strength testing and important measures of performance.

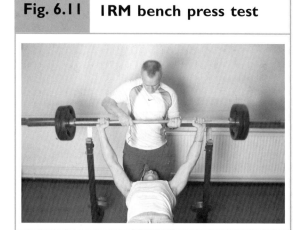

Fig. 6.11 1RM bench press test

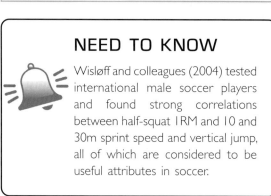

NEED TO KNOW

Wisløff and colleagues (2004) tested international male soccer players and found strong correlations between half-squat 1RM and 10 and 30m sprint speed and vertical jump, all of which are considered to be useful attributes in soccer.

Strength testing with machines

Due to the availability of testing equipment, resistance machines are often used for strength testing. Testing procedures used to measure strength with resistance machines are similar to free weight testing procedures but testing can be performed more quickly as the weight increments are often easier to adjust and there is usually less experience or familiarity required on the part of the subject being tested.

Even though the external resistance is constant in the case of both machine and free weight testing methods, strength measurements may vary between different machines (same type of machine but different manufacturer) by a greater extent than free weights. This is because of the design of the machine and quite often the difference in mechanical efficiency (this can be due to many factors such as number of cams, friction between surfaces, type of cord or belt used etc).

Another difference between machine and free weight strength testing is that spotters are not generally required when testing with resistance machines. Also the reduced skill required to use the machines is sometimes considered more conducive to assessing pure strength more accurately than free weights.

Similarly to strength testing with free weights, the body position of the subject during machine testing is very important as far as reliability is concerned. Start positions during exercises such as machine bench press or machine squats have

been shown to affect the measures of strength values obtained.

It is quite common that with many resistance-machines the weight increments are more limited than those of free weights. This can be a potential disadvantage as typical resistance machine increments of 5kg may be too great for the determination of true strength values.

One of the main advantages of using resistance machines for strength-testing purposes is generally considered to be the linear nature of the movement of the subject when performing the test. On the other hand, one of the main limitations of resistance-machine strength testing is the lack of coordination required on the part of the subject being tested. This is considered to be unlike typical movements performed in sporting situations.

Table 6.3	Normative values for squat strength (1-RM kg/kg bodyweight)				
	Age (yr)				
Rating	20–29	30–39	40–49	50–59	>59
MEN					
Excellent	>2.07	>1.87	>1.75	>1.65	>1.55
Good	2.00–2.07	1.80–1.87	1.70–1.75	1.60–1.65	1.50–1.55
Average	1.83–1.99	1.63–1.79	1.56–1.69	1.46–1.59	1.37–1.49
Fair	1.65–1.82	1.55–1.62	1.50–1.55	1.40–1.45	1.31–1.36
Poor	<1.65	<1.55	<1.50	<1.40	<1.31
WOMEN					
Excellent	>1.62	>1.41	>1.31	>1.25	>1.14
Good	1.54–1.62	1.35–1.41	1.26–1.31	1.13–1.25	1.08–1.14
Average	1.35–1.53	1.20–1.34	1.12–1.25	0.99–1.12	0.92–1.07
Fair	1.26–1.34	1.13–1.19	1.06–1.11	0.86–0.98	0.85–0.91
Poor	<1.26	<1.13	<1.06	<0.86	<0.85

Table 6.4	Norm values for bench press strength (1-RM kg/kg bodyweight)				
	Age (yr)				
Rating	20–29	30–39	40–49	50–59	>59
MEN					
Excellent	>1.26	>1.08	>0.97	>0.86	>0.78
Good	1.17–1.25	1.01–1.07	0.91–0.96	0.81–0.85	0.74–0.77
Average	0.97–1.16	0.86–1.00	0.78–0.90	0.70–0.80	0.64–0.73
Fair	0.88–0.96	0.79–0.85	0.72–0.77	0.65–0.69	0.60–0.63
Poor	<0.87	<0.78	<0.71	<0.64	<0.59
WOMEN					
Excellent	>0.78	>0.66	>0.61	>0.54	>0.55
Good	0.72–0.77	0.62–0.65	0.57–0.60	0.51–0.53	0.51–0.54
Average	0.59–0.71	0.53–0.61	0.48–0.56	0.43–0.50	0.41–0.50
Fair	0.53–0.58	0.49–0.52	0.44–0.47	0.40–0.42	0.37–0.40
Poor	<0.52	<0.48	<0.43	<0.39	<0.36

Source: Tables adapted from American College of Sports Medicine (1988) *Guidelines for Exercise Testing and Prescription Resource Manual.*

Muscular endurance

As with muscular strength, muscular endurance (or 'local muscular endurance') is generally considered to be an important component of fitness, especially in many sports where large forces have to be applied repetitively, such as rowing (where up to 200 repetitions or strokes will be performed over a six-minute period).

As with defining muscular strength, it is also difficult to agree on a single definition of muscular endurance. It is often described as *'the ability of a muscle or muscle group to perform repeated contractions against a resistance over a period of time'* and is generally associated with resistance training using relatively low intensity (weight) and high repetitions. However, a more generally accepted definition of local muscular endurance could be stated as *'the number of repetitions to failure of a specific exercise performed using a certain resistance'.*

In many types of muscular endurance test, it is the subject's own body mass that provides the resistance (curl-up and press-up test), as opposed to free weights or resistance machines providing the resistance.

When performing endurance tests using free weights, the resistance is usually determined as a percentage of 1RM, for example 60 per cent or 80 per cent of 1RM. If the subject being tested is strength training on a regular basis, it is important that 1RM is assessed frequently to ensure that the test weight is an accurate percentage of the current 1RM for the subject.

Example: For an individual with a 1RM bench press of 75kg, 80 per cent of 1RM will be 60kg before training. If however after eight weeks of resistance training the new 1RM is 82.5kg, 80 per cent of 1RM is now 66kg. In other words, the training weight needs to increase.

In this particular example, performing a muscular endurance test with the 60kg weight will more likely result in a greater number of repetitions simply due to an increase in strength rather than to increased muscular endurance. For this reason, it is recommended to use the 1RM values obtained at the start of the training period in order to determine percentage of 1RM loads to be used, and then to reassess the load at the start of the next training period (the training period depends on the subject and the type of training).

The number of repetitions that the coach or instructor can expect to be performed during endurance testing varies depending on the particular exercise. However, repetitions can typically range from 6 to 20 for 80 per cent of 1RM, 11 to 45 for 60 per cent of 1RM, and 20 to 80 for 40 per cent of 1RM.

Although there are many local muscular endurance testing methods available for coaches and instructors, some of the more popular and easy to administer include the curl-up test, the press-up test and the chin-up test. As mentioned earlier, these types of endurance test rely on bodyweight as opposed to an external resistance.

Curl-up test

This is an easy to administer test that uses body-weight rather than an external resistance.

Required resources

Flat surface and mat.

Testing method

1. The subject lies on the mat with the knees bent, feet flat on the floor, and the hands resting on the thighs (see figure 6.12a).
2. Curl up slowly using the abdominal muscles and slide the hands up the thighs until the finger-tips touch the kneecaps (see figure 6.12b).
3. Return slowly to the starting position.
4. The feet are not to be held and a complete curl-up should take three seconds.
5. Repeat as many curl-ups as possible at this rate.

Analysis

Compare the results with those of previous tests or use the normative valves in tables 6.5a and b. With appropriate training between tests, analysis should indicate an improvement in muscular endurance.

Classification

Fig. 6.12 (a) Curl-up start point

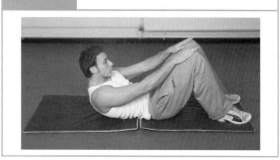

Fig. 6.12 (b) Curl-up end point

Table 6.5a	Normative values for male curl-ups			
Age	Excellent	Good	Fair	Poor
<35	60	45	30	15
35–44	50	40	25	10
>44	40	25	15	5

Table 6.5b	Normative values for female curl-ups			
Age	Excellent	Good	Fair	Poor
<35	50	40	25	10
35–44	40	25	15	6
>44	30	15	10	4

Press-up test

This is considered to be an easy-to-administer test that uses bodyweight rather than an external resistance. The test requires little in the way of equipment and is often used to assess muscular endurance for groups or teams.

Required resources

A flat surface and a mat.

Testing method

1. Lie on the mat, hands shoulder-width apart, and fully extend the arms (figure 6.13a).
2. Lower the body until the elbows reach 90° (mid position) as in figure 6.13b.
3. Return to the starting position with the arms fully extended.
4. The push-up action should be continuous with no rest periods.
5. Record the total number of full-body press-ups completed by the subject before fatigue.

Fig. 6.13 **(a) Press-up test start position**

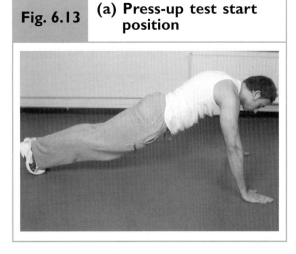

Fig. 6.13 **(b) Press-up test mid position**

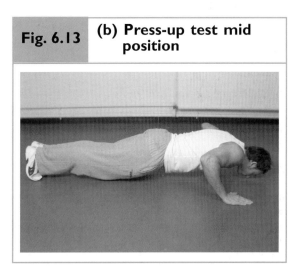

Modified press-up test

It is sometimes the case that subjects are not able to complete full press-ups (or can only do very few); therefore, for those subjects who have relatively weak upper body strength, the modified press-up test can be used. The test is then performed as follows:

1. Lie on the mat, hands shoulder-width apart, bent knee position, and fully extend the arms (figure 6.14a).
2. Lower the upper body until the elbows reach 90° (mid position as in figure 6.14b).
3. Return to the starting position with the arms fully extended.
4. The push-up action should be continuous with no rest periods.
5. Record the total number of modified press-ups completed by the subject before fatigue.

Analysis

Analysis of the results can be done by comparing them with the results of previous tests as with the sit-up test. It is expected that, with appropriate training between tests, the analysis would indicate an improvement in the subject's press-up muscular endurance.

Classification

The normative values in tables 6.6a and 6.6b are the test standards commonly used to

assess press up performance for both full-body and modified press-ups. These values relate to age.

Fig. 6.14 (a) **Modified press-up test start position**

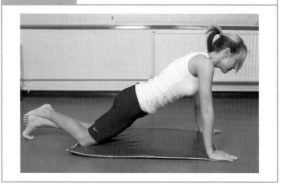

Fig. 6.14 (b) **Modified press-up test mid position**

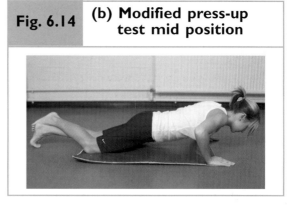

Table 6.6a	Normative values for full-body press-ups				
Age	Excellent	Good	Average	Fair	Poor
20–29	>54	45–54	35–44	20–34	<20
30–39	>44	35–44	25–34	15–24	<15
40–49	>39	30–39	20–29	12–19	<12
50–59	>34	25–34	15–24	8–14	<8
>59	>29	20–29	10–19	5–9	<5

Table 6.6b	Normative values for modified press-ups				
Age	Excellent	Good	Average	Fair	Poor
20–29	>48	34–48	17–33	6–16	<6
30–39	>39	25–39	12–24	4–11	<4
40–49	>34	20–34	8–19	3–7	<3
50–59	>29	15–29	6–14	2–5	<2
>59	>19	5–19	3–4	1–2	<1

Chin-up test

This is an easy-to-administer test that uses body-weight rather than an external resistance.

Required resources

A fixed bar with sufficient clearance. A lat pull-down machine may help in warming up and preparing for the test.

Testing method

1. Subject should warm up and gently stretch shoulders and latissimus dorsi.
2. If a lat pull-down machine is available, they should perform 8–10 repetitions of lat pull-downs at approximately 33 per cent of 1RM.
3. Gently stretch shoulders and latissimus dorsi.
4. Subject should perform six repetitions of lat pull-downs at approximately 65 per cent of 1RM.
5. The subject should adopt an overhand grip on the fixed bar, shoulder-width apart, achieving full arm extension.
6. Knees should always remain bent to 90° and body near-vertical throughout.
7. As many chin-ups as possible should be performed without stopping, raising the chin above the bar and fully extending the arms.
8. Load may be increased through the use of a weighted belt.

Analysis

For elite rugby union players, forwards should aim to complete over 10 repetitions, and backs over 15 repetitions (Tong and Wiltshire 2007). As many as 24 ± 11 repetitions have been achieved on average by Australian international outside backs (Jenkins and Raeburn 2000).

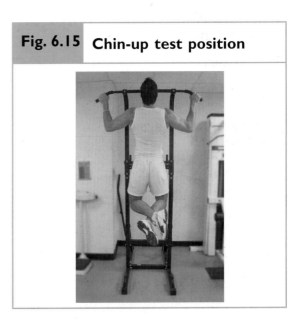

Fig. 6.15 Chin-up test position

Muscular endurance assessed by isokinetic dynamometry

Isokinetic dynamometry, as described previously (see page 129), can be used to give an assessment of local muscular endurance. Parameters frequently measured include:

- Fatigue index, which is the percentage decrease in peak torque.
- Percentage decrease in peak torque over a 30- 60- or 120-second period.
- Time until torque falls to 50 per cent of peak value.
- Number of repetitions performed until torque falls to 50 per cent of peak value.
- Ratio of work performed in the first third of the bout to the last third of the bout.

One of the advantages of this technique is the controlled nature of the test; however, disadvantages are the expense involved in accessing the equipment and the practicalities of its use compared to standard field testing. Therefore the protocol for this type of testing will not be covered within this book.

Further reading

Aagaard, P., Simonsen, E., Andersen, J., Magnusson, P. & Dyhre-Poulsen, P. (2002) 'Increased rate of force development and neural drive of human skeletal muscle following resistance training'. *Journal of Applied Physiology*, 93: pp. 1318-26

Abernethy, P. & Wilson, G. (2007) 'Introduction to the assessment of strength and power'. In Gore, C. (ed.) *Physiological Tests for Elite Athletes*, Champaign, Illinois: Human Kinetics, pp. 147-50

American College of Sports Medicine (1998) 'Position Stand: Exercise and physical activity for older adults'. *Medicine and Science in Sport and Exercise*, 30: pp. 992-1008

American College of Sports Medicine (1998) 'Postion Statement: The recommended quantity and quality of exercise for developing and maintaining cardiorespiratory and muscular fitness and flexibility in healthy adults'. *Medicine and Science in Sport and Exercise*, 30(6): pp. 975-91

American College of Sports Medicine. (2002) Kraemer, W. J., Writing Group Chairman. 'Position Stand: Progression models in resistance training for healthy adults'. *Medicine and Science in Sports and Exercise*, 34: pp. 364-80

Bachele, T. (ed.) (1994) *Essentials of Strength Training and Conditioning*, Champaign, Illinois: Human Kinetics

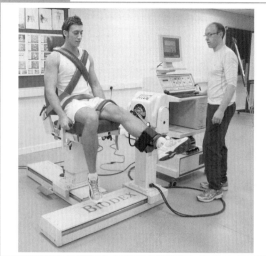

Fig. 6.16 | **Typical isokinetic dynamometry testing**

Baltzopoulos, V. & Gleeson, N. P. (2001) 'Skeletal muscle function'. In Eston, R. & Reilly, T. (eds.), *Kinanthropometry and Exercise Physiology Laboratory Manual: Tests, procedures and data,* 2nd edn, (Volume 2: Exercise physiology), London, UK: Routledge, pp. 1-35

Benjamin, H. J. & Glow, K. M. (2003) 'Strength training for children and adolescents'. *Physical Sports Medicine,* 31: pp. 19-27

Blimkie, C. J. R. (1992) 'Resistance training during pre- and early puberty: Efficacy, trainability, mechanisms and persistence'. *Canadian Journal of Sports Science,* 17: pp. 264-79

Blimkie, C. J. R. & Sale, D. G. (1998) 'Strength development and trainability during childhood'. In van Praagh, E. (ed.) *Pediatric anaerobic performance,* Champaign, Illinois: Human Kinetics, pp. 193-224

Braith, R., Graves, J., Leggett, S. & Pollock, M. (1993) 'Effect of training on the relationship between maximal and submaximal strength'. *Medicine and Science in Sports and Exercise,* 25: pp. 132-8

Brzycki, M. (1993) 'Strength testing – Predicting a one-rep max from reps-to-fatigue'. *JOPERD,* January: pp. 88-90

Calder, A., Chilibeck, P., Webber, C. & Sale, D. (1994) 'Comparison of whole and split weight training routines in young women'. *Canadian Journal of Applied Physiology,* 19: pp. 185-99

Carpinelli, R. & Otto, R. (1998) 'Strength training: Single versus multiple sets'. *Sports Medicine,* 26: pp. 73-84

Clark, H. C. (1966) *Muscular Strength and Endurance in Man,* New York, New York: Prentice-Hall

Coldwells, A., Atkinson, G. & Reilly, T. (1994) 'Sources of variation in back and leg dynamometry'. *Ergonomics,* 37: pp. 79-86

Cosgrove, L. & Mayhew, J. (1997) 'A modified YMCA bench press test to predict strength in adult women'. *IAHPERD Journal* [online periodical] accessed March 2009, http://www.iowaahperd.org/journal/j97s_bench.html

Coulson, M. & Archer, D. (2008) *Fitness Professionals: The Advanced Fitness Instructor's Handbook,* London, UK: A&C Black

Davis, J. A., Brewer, J. & Atkin, D. (1992) 'Preseason physiological characteristics of English first and second division soccer players'. *Journal of Sports Science,* 10: pp. 541-7

Fatouros, I. G., Jamurtas, A. Z., Leontsini, D., Taxildaris, K., Aggelousis, N., Kostopoulos, N. & Buckenmeyer, P. (2000) 'Evaluation of plyometric exercise training, weight training, and their combination on vertical jumping performance and leg strength'. *Journal of Strength and Conditioning Research,* 14: pp. 470-6

Feigenbaum, M. & Pollock, M. (1997) 'Strength training: Rationale for current guidelines for adult fitness programs'. *Physician and Sports Medicine,* 25: pp. 44-64

Fleck, S. J. & Kraemer, W. J. (2004) *Designing Resistance Training Programmes,* 2nd edn, Champaign, Illinois: Human Kinetics, pp. 199-216

Folland, J. P., Irish, C. S., Roberts, J. C., Tarr, J. E. & Jones, D. A. (2002) 'Fatigue as a stimulus for strength gains during resistance training'. *British Journal of Sports Medicine*, 36: pp. 370-4

Jenkins, D. & Raeburn, G. (2000) 'Protocols for the physiological assessment of rugby union players'. In Gore, C. (ed.) *Physiological Tests for Elite Athletes*, Champaign, Illinois: Human Kinetics, pp. 327-33

Johnson, C. (1994) 'Elastic strength development'. *Athletics Coach*, 28: pp. 5-7

Kaelin, M. E., Swank, A. M., Adams, K. J., Barnard, K. L., Berning, J. M. & Green, A. (1999) 'Cardiopulmonary responses, muscle soreness, and injury during the one repetition maximum assessment in pulmonary rehabilitation patients'. *Journal of Cardiopulmonary Rehabilitation*, 19: pp. 366-72

Knapik, J. J., et al (1983) 'Angular specificity and test mode specificity of isometric and isokinetic strength training'. *Journal of Orthopedic Sports Physical Therapy*, 5: pp. 58-65

Kraemer, W. J. & Fleck, S. J. (2007) *Optimizing Strength Training: Designing nonlinear periodization workouts*, Champaign, Illinois: Human Kinetics

Lander, J. (1985) 'Maximum based on reps'. *National Strength and Conditioning Association Journal*, 6: pp. 60-1

Leong, B., et al (1999) 'Maximal motor unit discharge rates in quadriceps muscles of older weight lifters'. *Medicine and Science in Sports and Exercise*, 31: pp. 1638-44

Logan, P., Fornasiero, D., Abernethy, P. & Lynch, K. (2000) 'Protocols for the assessment of isoinertial strength'. In Gore, C. (ed.) *Physiological Tests for Elite Athletes*, Champaign, Illinois: Human Kinetics, pp. 200-22

Mayhew, J. L., Ware, J. S., Bemben, M. G., Wilt, B., Ward, T. E., Farris, B., Juraszek, J. & Slovak, J. P. (1999) 'The NFL-225 test as a measure of bench press strength in college football players'. *Journal of Strength and Conditioning Research*, 13: pp. 130-4

Pavone, E. & Moffat, M. (1985) 'Isometric torque of the quadriceps femoris after concentric, eccentric and isometric training'. *Archives of Physical Medical Rehabilitation*, 66: pp. 168-70

Ploutz-Snyder, L. L., Giamis, E. L., Formikell, M. & Rosenbaum, A. E. (2001) 'Resistance training reduces susceptibility to eccentric exercise induced muscle dysfunction in older women'. *Journals of the Gerontology Series A: Biological and Medical Sciences*, 56A: B384-B390.

Poliquin, C. & King, I. (1992) 'Theory and methodology of training'. *Sports Coach*, April–June

Poliquin, C. (1992) *Theory and Methodology of Strength Training: ASCA Level 2 Resource Manual*, ASCA: Australian Coaching Council

Rantanen, T., Guralnik, J. M., Foley, D., Masaki, K., Leveille, S., Curb, J. D. & White, L. (1999) 'Midlife hand grip strength as a predictor of old age disability'. *Journal of the American Medical Association,* 281: pp. 558-60

Reynolds, J. M., Gordon, T. J. & Robergs, R. A. (2006) 'Prediction of one repetition maximum strength from multiple repetition maximum testing and anthropometry'. *Journal of Strength and Conditioning Research*, 20: pp. 584-92

Sale, D. G. (1986) 'Neural Adaptations in strength and power training'. In Jones, Norman L. *Human Muscle Power*, Champaign, Illinois: Human Kinetics

Sale, D. G. (1988) 'Neural adaptation to resistance training'. *Medicine and Science in Sports and Exercise*, 20: pp. S135-S145

Sewell, L. P. & Lander, J. E. (1991) 'The effects of rest on maximal efforts in the squat and bench press'. *Journal of Applied Sports Science Research*, 5: pp. 96-9

Starkey, D. B., Pollock, M. L., Ishida, Y., Welsch, M. A., Brechue, W. F., Graves, J. E. & Feigenbaum, M. S. (1996) 'Effect of resistance training volume on strength and muscle thickness'. *Medicine and Science in Sports and Exercise*, 28: pp. 1311-20

Steindler, A. (1935) *Mechanics of Normal and Pathological Locomotion in Man*, Baltimore, Maryland: Thomas

Stone, M. H., Fleck, S. J., Kraemer, W. J. & Triplett, N. T. (1991) 'Health and performance-related potential of resistance training'. *Sports Medicine*, 11: pp. 210-31

Syddall, H., Cooper, C., Martin, F., Briggs, R., Aihie Sayer, A. (2003) 'Is grip strength a useful single marker of frailty?' *Age and Ageing*, 32: pp. 650-6

Tong, R. J. & Wiltshire, H. D. (2007) 'Rugby Union'. In Winter, E. M., Jones, A. M., Davison, R. C., Bromley, P. & Mercer, T. (eds.) *Sport and Exercise Science Testing Guidelines: The British Association of Sport and Exercise Sciences Guide. Volume I: Sport Testing*, London and New York: Routledge, pp. 327-33

Voight, M. & Klausen, K. (1990) 'Changes in muscle strength and speed of an unloaded movement after various training programmes'. *European Journal of Applied Physiology*, 60: pp. 370-76

Wardle, H. & Wilson, G. (1996) 'Practical strength programming training tips for athletes: What works'. *Strength Conditioning Coach*, 4: pp. 3-5

Weir, J. P., Housh, T. J., Weir, L. L. & Johnson, G. O. (1995) 'Effects of unilateral isometric strength training on joint angle specificity and cross-training'. *European Journal of Applied Physiology*, 70: pp. 337-43

Wilson, G. (2007) 'Limitations on the use of isometric assessment in athletic assessment'. In Gore, C. (ed.) *Physiological Tests for Elite Athletes*, Champaign, Illinois: Human Kinetics, pp. 151-4

Wisløff, U., Castagna, C., Helgerud, J., Jones, R. & Hoff, J. (2004) 'Strong correlation of maximal squat strength with sprint performance and vertical jump height in elite soccer players'. *British Journal of Sports Medicine*, 38: pp. 285-8

Wrigley, T. & Strauss, G. (2000) 'Strength assessment by isokinetic dynamometry'. In Gore, C. (ed.) *Physiological Tests for Elite Athletes*, Champaign, Illinois: Human Kinetics, pp. 155-99

Young, W. B. (1995) 'Laboratory strength assessment of athletes'. *New Studies in Athletics*, 10(1): pp. 86-96

SPEED AND AGILITY TESTING

7

OBJECTIVES

After completing this chapter you should be able to:

1 Explain the terms 'speed', 'reaction speed', and 'acceleration'.

2 Identify the components of sprint speed.

3 List a range of sports and events for which speed is a vital component and discuss the importance of various speed components in relation to those sports or events.

4 List and discuss the various positive and negative factors that contribute to speed development.

5 Explain the terms 'stride length' and 'stride rate' and how they can affect sprint speed.

6 Understand the cost implications offset by accuracy benefits of using electronic measuring devices.

7 Explain the use of different protocols and the effectiveness of speed, balance and agility testing methods.

8 Recognise how sprint testing is dictated by the event or sport of the subject.

9 Define the term 'agility' and the related components known as 'programmed and random agility'.

Speed

In relation to training and assessment of athletes, speed may be thought of in two ways. One is the speed of an initial reaction to a stimulus. Another way is the speed of the body in any direction along the ground.

Speed along the ground is a parameter with many components that are often trained for separately. These components, such as balance, strength and efficiency of movement, should be trained for and tested not only in a linear or forward direction, but also in a multi-directional way, which will enable athletes to access optimal preparation for a multitude of sports and activities.

Activities that increase the ability of the body to react to a variety of stimuli should also be included within the training programme (and tested for), as these will assist in improving decision-making tasks within a sports environment.

Sprinting, and therefore speed, at maximum or near-maximum effort over various distances is important for many track and field events. Track sprint events may include the 100 metres, 110 metre hurdles, 200 metres, 400 metres, 400 metre hurdles, and 4×100 and 4×400 metre relays (and it could be argued that all middle-distance events have an important requirement for sprint speed). Sprint speed is also a crucial component of certain field events such as the long jump, triple jump, pole vault, hammer and javelin.

Reaction and the initial rate of force development are considered to be important for events such as combat sports, while acceleration and the ability to reproduce sprint speed can be considered important for participants in court games such as basketball and tennis. In some activities, such as combat sports, racquet games and throwing events, upper-limb speed is as important as lower-limb speed.

Although speed is a complex construct, for the purpose of this book speed is broken down into several components as can be seen in figure 7.1.

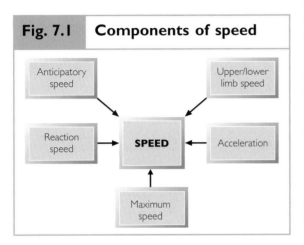

Fig. 7.1 Components of speed

In many sports, improvements in reaction speed or acceleration are often more appropriate than improvements in maximum speed. Athletes might not reach maximum sprinting speed until they have run 50–60 metres, for example, and, in sports such as soccer and Australian Rules football, distances of about 10–20 metres are the most common 'sprint'

distances covered. Therefore, speed testing methods for these types of sport (normally team multi-sprint sports) should have protocols that focus on distances typically covered within them. Specificity of testing also applies to sports such as boxing and martial arts, in which upper- and lower-limb speed is an essential component of the sport and should be tested for, whereas in track events, such as 100 to 400 metre sprinting, maximal sprint speed (and maintenance of that maximal speed) becomes an important factor for testing purposes.

Factors contributing to speed development

Due to the complex nature and many integral components of speed, there are many training methods commonly used to affect sprint speed and as a result there are also a great number of testing methods. If specific factors are identified that could have a potentially positive effect on sprint speed performance, it follows that testing methods can be employed to investigate each of these factors. Conversely, there are also specific factors that could negatively affect sprint speed performance and these factors could also be tested for. Table 7.1 gives a simplistic overview of the positive and negative factors that could potentially

Table 7.1	Potential factors affecting sprint speed performance
Positive factors	**Negative factors**
Muscular strength	Excess body fat
Power	Fatigue
Flexibility	Low cardiovascular fitness levels
% of fast-twitch fibres	Technique
Neuromuscular firing rates	
Technique	

contribute to overall sprint performance; however, some of the testing methods (such as percentage of fast-twitch fibres) should only be carried out by suitably qualified people (those with clinical experience) in a laboratory environment and the results are of limited use for athletes.

You can argue about the contribution of both positive and negative factors to sprint speed performance, but most coaches would agree that an improvement in all of the positive factors would benefit the athlete's performance. From the coach's or tester's perspective, individual positive and negative factors should be regularly monitored and measured, and correlated against results of specific speed performance to help identify those factors that might be positively or negatively contributing.

Stride length and stride rate

One of the main areas often considered by coaches to contribute to potential improvements in speed performance is *stride length* and/or *stride rate.*

Stride length can be described simply as the distance (normally in metres) between consecutive strides when walking or running. Stride rate is the total number of strides taken over a period of one second.

Stride length can be assessed by measuring the distance covered over a certain number of strides using normal sprinting technique. You may need an assistant to help you identify the start and finish of the distance covered. For example, a sprinter covering 40.5 metres with 18 strides has an average stride length of 2.25 metres.

Stride rate can be measured by timing a sprint and counting the number of strides completed. Continuing the above example, if the 40.5 metres are covered in 5.0 seconds, then the stride rate is 3.6 strides per second.

Anecdotally, many athletes and coaches concentrate initially on improving stride length only to find that both stride rate and speed can

be adversely affected, resulting in a subsequent decrease of both. It is perhaps more effective to focus on trying to improve the stride rate of the athlete first, because this often has the effect of increasing the power in the leg muscles, which in turn increases the stride length.

Coaches and athletes often assume that an individual stride length can be calculated as a consequence of the height of the athlete. Even though this is true to a certain extent, there is a disparity in the research as to the exact relationship between these two variables (subject height and stride length).

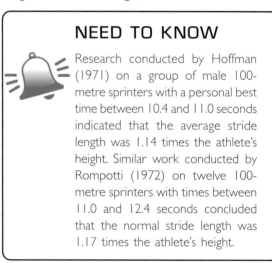

NEED TO KNOW

Research conducted by Hoffman (1971) on a group of male 100-metre sprinters with a personal best time between 10.4 and 11.0 seconds indicated that the average stride length was 1.14 times the athlete's height. Similar work conducted by Rompotti (1972) on twelve 100-metre sprinters with times between 11.0 and 12.4 seconds concluded that the normal stride length was 1.17 times the athlete's height.

Despite the differences in abilities of the athletes tested in each group of the highlighted examples, the results can be seen to be fairly similar. However, further research work conducted by Atwater (1979) on twenty-three 100-metre sprinters, with times varying between 9.9 and 10.4 seconds, concluded that the average stride length was actually 1.35 times the athlete's height.

One of the reasons for the differences in the results could have been that the testing carried out by Hoffman and Rompotti was conducted on cinder-surface tracks, whereas the testing carried out by Atwater was conducted on synthetic-surface tracks.

Using Atwater's results, a six-foot athlete (1.8 metres) can be calculated to have an average stride length of 2.5 metres.

Regardless of the reasons for differences in the research, the variation highlights that stride length is difficult to estimate based on the height of the athlete.

Sprint testing

Testing for sprint speed usually involves subjects running linear distances of 20–50 metres. The testing surface can vary but should be kept consistent in terms of follow-up testing, and specific to the associated sport or event.

A stopwatch is cheap to use, but measurement will be flawed due to human error incurred at the start and end of the test. For accuracy, use light-gates (electronic timing devices) but these can be expensive to purchase and maintain. A full set of Bower timing gates costs in the region of £1,000.

The most variable test surface is grass as weather conditions can greatly affect the hardness and hence sprint speed.

Standing starts tend to be the more commonly used; however, flying starts may be more valid for team sports. Distances can also be made specific to the sport, so for cricketers, the distance between wickets (17.7 metres) is used for sprint testing. Similarly for baseball players, the one or two-base sprint test is frequently used. These baseball tests cover distances of 17.9 metres (one base) and 35.8 metres (two bases), taking either 3 or 6 seconds, respectively. For athletes in team sports, the distances covered are rarely in excess of 20 metres and so testing for speed over 5, 10 and 20 metres is frequently performed (table 7.2). Exceptions are rugby union or rugby league where 10- and 40-metre distances are often timed. For track sprinters, the distances covered should be relative to the events performed. Highly trained or elite-level sprinters usually reach their individual maximal speed at distances of approximately 50–60 metres, whereas in less trained individuals, maximal speed is normally reached after approximately 30 metres. The maximal speed phase of sprinting (compared to other phases of speed) plays only a minor role in many team sports.

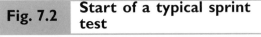

Fig. 7.2 Start of a typical sprint test

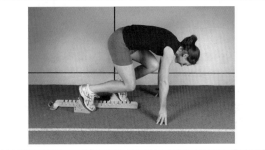

Required resources

Stopwatch (or light gates), a 20–50 metre straight track or field, tape measure.

Testing method

1 Mark the start and finish of the distance being tested.
2 Subject lines up (sprint or standing start) on the start line of the straight track.
3 The tester gives the command to go and starts the stopwatch at the same time.
4 The tester should record the time for the subject to complete the distance.
5 Repeat the test several times and record the fastest time. Allow the subject complete recovery between sprints. The subject can have as many efforts as they choose.

Analysis

Analysis of the results involves comparing them with the results of previous tests. Table 7.3, however, gives the speed classification for adults for a 30-metre sprint.

Table 7.2	Elite team-sports athletes' 5, 10, 20, 30 and 40m sprint times				
Sport (gender)	5m sprint time (s)	10m sprint time (s)	20m sprint time (s)	30m sprint time (s)	40m sprint time (s)
Soccer (M) English		1.71		4.14	
Soccer (M) Australian	1.03	1.74	3.04		
Soccer (F) Australian	1.11	1.91	3.29		
Field hockey (M)		1.86	3.18		
Field hockey (F)		2.00			
Rugby union (M) Forward		1.80 (position not specified)	3.10 (position not specified)	4.50	6.30
Rugby union (M) Back		1.80 (position not specified)	3.10 (position not specified)	4.30	5.80
Rugby league (M) Forward		2.00	3.10		5.60
Rugby league (M) Back		1.90	2.90		5.30
Basketball (M)	1.05	1.75	3.00		
Basketball (F)	1.20	2.05	3.50		

Table 7.3	Speed rating for adults for a 30-metre sprint (values in seconds)				
Gender	Excellent	Above average	Average	Below average	Poor
Male	<4.0	4.0–4.2	4.3–4.4	4.5–4.6	>4.6
Female	<4.5	4.5–4.6	4.7–4.8	4.9–5.0	>5.0

Repeated sprint test (RST)

Team sports tend to be highly intense and intermittent in nature, consisting of bouts of high-intensity work followed by extended periods of low-intensity work (to recover from the high-intensity work). The ability to perform and recover from repeated sprints is vital for sports players. It must be remembered however that the recovery durations can vary widely during a match. For instance, following a sprint for a loose ball, a player might have to sprint again immediately to cover an opponent's attack.

Coaches in team sports frequently assess their players' ability to perform repeated sprints. Many of the repeated sprint tests that have been developed have been shown to be very reliable, with a typical error of measurement of approximately 1 per cent or less. Be aware, however, that subjects often pace themselves during repeated sprint tests, invalidating the results, particularly if there are a large number of repetitions to perform. This has been evidenced by the authors on many testing occasions.

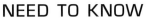

NEED TO KNOW

Psotta and Bunc (2003) found that soccer players' sprint speed on their first sprint was 5 per cent slower than their 20-metre sprint time, indicating that they were using a pacing strategy.

One way to avoid this particular problem is to get all subjects to perform a maximal sprint over the chosen test distance before beginning the actual repeated sprint test. If the subjects are more than 2 per cent slower than when performing their first sprint, this may indicate that they are pacing themselves.

NEED TO KNOW

Sometimes players that are being tested pace themselves, as they are aware that they have, for example, ten sprints to perform and hence will not go 'all out' from the first sprint, as it will be more painful.

Encourage subjects, therefore, to work maximally for each sprint and avoid pacing themselves. The choices of distances, direction or recovery times will be influenced by the sport and possibly even by position within a sport. The distances covered in repeated sprint tests vary between 20 and 40 metres, the number of repetitions varies between 6 and 18 and the recovery time varies between 15 and 25 seconds. Recovery duration is important, as it has been shown that no fatigue is evident when performing 15 sprints of 5–6 seconds duration with recovery durations of 120 seconds. This lack of fatigue is probably related to the time course of recovery of phosphocreatine (see chapter 2) among other things. When the recovery was reduced to either 30 or 60 seconds, fatigue occurred after the 5th and 11th sprint, respectively. The degree of fatigue during repeated sprint tests is related to the aerobic fitness of the subjects. More aerobically fit subjects tend to have a lower fatigue index than those subjects who are less fit. Typical research comparisons of athletes in team sports often show greater peak-power outputs (or sprint speeds), but greater fatigue rates than athletes from endurance sports.

Multiple sprint test
Required resources

Stopwatch (or light gates), a 20-metre straight track or field, tape measure, cones.

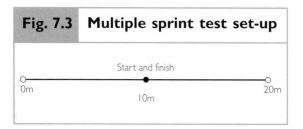

| Fig. 7.3 | Multiple sprint test set-up |

Start and finish

0m ———————————————— 20m
10m

Testing method

1 Measure out a 20-metre course accurately and mark with cones at 0, 10 and 20 metres.
2 Start subjects at the midway point (10 metres) and run to the 0-metre point, across to the 20-metre point and finally back to the midway point where they started (the total distance covered per sprint will be 40 metres).
3 The tester gives the command to go and starts the stopwatch at the same time. Subjects are to start sprinting at the exact moment of this command.
4 Record sprint time. Allow 20 seconds rest (time this with a stopwatch) and repeat sprint again.
5 Subjects will perform eight sprints, each of which should be 'all out' and at maximal intensity if the results are to be useful.
6 Record the time for each of the eight sprints (for each subject), then calculate the fatigue index across the range of the eight sprints (see p. 155-6 for equations).

This test is commonly used with rugby union players, as the requirements for changes in direction are relevant to this and most team sports.

Running-based anaerobic sprint test (RAST)

The RAST was developed by researchers Draper and Whyte at the University of Wolverhampton and was designed to be similar to the Wingate anaerobic test (see chapter 8). Subjects are required to perform six 35-metre sprints with 10 seconds recovery between sprints (see figure 7.3). If timing gates are not used then there must be two timers (one on each start point as the subject will not have time to return to the first start point for the next sprint). The subject's body mass should be recorded before starting the test and the time for each sprint recorded. Using the following equations power output can be calculated:

$$Velocity = Distance / Time$$

$$Acceleration = Velocity / Time$$

$$Force = Mass \times Acceleration$$

$$Power = Force \times Velocity$$

It has been reported that power outputs of approximately 700W and calculated fatigue

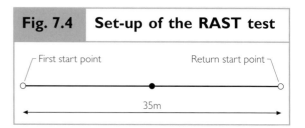

| Fig. 7.4 | Set-up of the RAST test |

First start point   Return start point

35m

indexes of 5–7 per cent have been observed on many occasions during running-based anaerobic sprint testing of 15 to 16-year-old male basketball players.

The intermittent anaerobic running test IAnRT test

The IAnRT is similar to the RAST but was designed for soccer players and developed by researchers in the Czech Republic. Subjects are required to complete ten maximal 20-metre sprints with 20 seconds recovery between sprints. The authors have found significant fatigue of subjects in sprints 8, 9 and 10 when conducting this test in the university laboratory reasonably on trained amateur soccer players.

The 6 × 30m RST with active recovery (field-hockey players)

This repeated sprint test involves sprinting 30 metres, decelerating rapidly to a walk, jogging around two cones placed 20 metres apart (takes between 12 and 13 seconds), and waiting for 5 seconds at the new start position before the next sprint (see figure 7.5). Subjects are timed

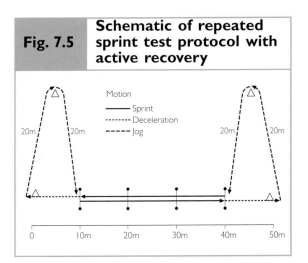

Fig. 7.5 | **Schematic of repeated sprint test protocol with active recovery**

Motion
—— Sprint
.... Deceleration
----- Jog

20m 20m   20m 20m

0   10m   20m   30m   40m   50m

at 10, 20 and 30 metres if timing gates are available.

This test is reliable and specifically designed for field hockey players, though it could be used for other team sports. The test measures are total sprint time and fatigue index. A study has shown that 30-metre times for highly trained Australian field hockey players decreased from 4.4 to 4.6 seconds over the six sprints.

Repeated Balsom run

This repeated sprint agility test was designed for soccer players and allows three subjects to be tested simultaneously.

Subjects perform five bouts of the Balsom run (described on page 162). The first subject starts running and a stopwatch is set. That subject's time is measured using timing gates. At 20 seconds on the stopwatch, the second subject starts sprinting and is timed. At 40 seconds, the third subject starts sprinting and is timed. At 60 seconds, the first athlete starts their second sprint and is timed. At 80 seconds, the second subject starts their second sprint and is timed. This is continued until all three subjects complete five sprints. Recovery between sprints is approximately 47–49 seconds. Total time for the five sprints is approximately 60 seconds in a sample of English Premier League soccer players. If no timing gates are available, an assistant is required to perform timings. Using fewer than three subjects at a time may make testing easier.

Fatigue index (FI)

A simple description of the fatigue index is normally given as the percentage decrease in power output from peak power output to minimal power output (measured during testing), and can be calculated by using either of the following equations:

$$FI = [(\text{peak speed} - \text{minimum speed})/\text{peak speed}] \times 100\%$$
or
$$FI = [(\text{slowest sprint time} - \text{fastest sprint time})/\text{slowest sprint time}] \times 100\%$$

Example: A hockey player performs six repeated 30-metre sprint tests. If the time for the fastest sprint was 4.4 seconds and the time for the slowest sprint was 4.6 seconds, the sprint speeds are therefore 6.81m.s^{-1} (30 divided by 4.4) and 6.52m.s^{-1} (30 divided by 4.6). The fatigue index can then be calculated as follows:

Using the equation $FI = [(\text{peak speed} - \text{minimum speed})/\text{peak speed}] \times 100\%$:

$$FI = [(6.81 - 6.52)/6.81] \times 100\% = 4.3\%$$

Or using the second equation:

$$FI = [(4.6 - 4.4)/4.6] \times 100\% = 4.3\% \text{ also}$$

Note: Some researchers question the reliability of the fatigue index measure and prefer to use the average sprint speed as a measure of performance.

Agility

The scientific research community has no specific definition of agility. In a sporting context, however, agility often refers to the ability to stop, start and change the direction of movement while maintaining the control of that movement.

One proposed definition of agility is *'a rapid whole-body movement with change of speed or direction in response to a stimulus'.*

It is also generally accepted that agility is made up of several discrete components such as balance, reaction or decision-making, coordination, technique, strength and power, which are all trainable components (some of these are referred to as cognitive components; see chapter 2).

Almost every sport and athletic event requires some form of ability on the part of the athlete to perform many agility-type movements. For the purpose of this book, however, and relating to testing protocol, agility can be divided into two discrete areas, *programmed* and *random* agility.

Programmed agility

If the movement pattern of an athlete is considered to be agile but does not involve the reaction to a stimulus at some time during the movement, it can be classified as *programmed agility*. Take the example of a tennis player being agile enough to reach a drop volley from the back of the court. The player has calculated the direction of the movement and has not needed to change this in response to an external stimulus (as long as the player 'reads' or anticipates any slice or spin placed on the ball).

Random agility

If the movement pattern of an athlete is considered to be agile and *does* involve the reaction to a stimulus, the movement can be classified as *random agility*. Take the example of a goalkeeper who reacts to a well-struck volley heading for the far corner of the goal but the ball then takes a deflection. After starting to move in one direction, the goalkeeper is agile enough to change body position quickly in order to make the save. Another example would be a ball-carrier in rugby who was trying to side-step opponents in a random manner depending on the position of the opposition and the nature of the move.

Balance

Balance can be described as *'the process by which individuals maintain equilibrium and move their bodies in a specific relationship to the environment'*. It has also been stated that the ability to balance is an automatic and unconscious process that allows individuals to resist the destabilising effect of gravity, and is essential for purposeful movement. Balance is generally considered to be a fundamental component of effective movement.

In any form of movement, balance is essential for effective foot placement, body control and reduction of 'centre of mass' movement, therefore balance may be described as control of the centre of mass.

There are several systems within the body that contribute to balance, namely the proprioception, visual and vestibular systems.

Proprioceptors are sensory receptors located about the body. They detect muscular tension, tension in tendons and ligaments, relative tension, and pressure on the skin (the body also has a range of other sensory receptors that detect balance). The ability to express balance and coordination is highly dependent on the effectiveness of the body's internal sensory receptors and proprioceptors. The brain also relies upon information from the eyes and the ears for balance purposes.

Through training these systems, the ability to perform balance skills can become more effective. The central nervous system becomes more able to interpret these messages and formulate the appropriate movement response.

The 'neural networks' within the central nervous system become more extensive, as more and more neural links are created through repetition of movement skills. When complex movement patterns are introduced, the requirements of balance are increased. The need to land, accelerate, change direction and decelerate, which is often found in speed- or agility-type movements, requires advanced balance skills.

Essentially balance can be categorised as either *static* or *dynamic*. In other words, static balance relates to balance in a fixed position, whereas dynamic balance relates to balance during motion.

Testing of balance can be carried out with athletic populations for the purpose of performance, or for populations such as the elderly for the purpose of function to prevent injury as a result of falls.

Balance testing

With recent advances in technology, laboratory methods of measuring balance have become more and more common. Force plates are used to assess postural sway while more technical equipment is now available to measure centre of gravity and postural alignment during static and dynamic movements. Due to the obvious cost implications of these methods, other more subjective tests have been devised and correlated for validity purposes. These types of test are inexpensive and normally just require the tester to make subjective ratings of balance performance. The stork stand test is commonly used as a static balance test whereas the bass dynamic test is often used to assess dynamic balance.

Stork stand test

One drawback of this test is that some subjects will be able to hold this position for long periods of time, so stop after one minute.

Testing method

1. The subject stands comfortably with both feet on the floor and with their hands on their hips.
2. The subject lifts one leg and places the toes of that foot against the knee of the other leg.
3. On command the subject then raises their heel to stand on the toes.
4. The stopwatch is started and the subject balances for as long as possible without letting either the heel touch the ground or the other foot move away from the knee. Repeat on the opposite leg.

Classification

Table 7.4 can be used to classify balance ability for 16 to 19-year-old males and females.

Tests of static balance used for special populations with potentially poor balance are similar to the stork test, but significantly safer and easier for elderly or infirm populations to perform. The tests involve the subjects maintaining balance when their base of support is reduced and eyes open or closed. The following stances are commonly used and

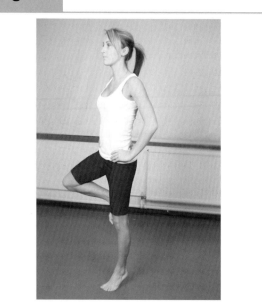

Fig. 7.6 **Stork stand test**

the duration of holding these positions is recorded.

- Feet touching, side by side.
- One foot moved half a length forwards.
- One foot in front of the other, heel to toe.

Table 7.4	Normative stork-stand to balance data for 16 to 19-year-olds (values in seconds)				
Gender	Excellent	Above average	Average	Below average	Poor
Male	>50	50–41	40–31	30–20	<20
Female	>30	30–23	22–16	15–10	<10

Bass dynamic test

This dynamic balance test requires subjects to complete a pattern, hopping and landing on a series of 10 marks placed on the floor (see figure 7.7). The direction in which the subject can begin the test (i.e. to the left or right) depends on leg dominance. Landing marks can be produced by using one-by-one inch pieces of marking tape. This test is reasonably easy to administer.

Required resources

Tape measure, flat surface, marking tape, stopwatch.

Testing method

1 The subject lines up at the start point.
2 The subject then leaps off the right foot and lands on the left foot (change this if going off the opposite foot).
3 On landing on each mark, the subject attempts to completely cover it with the metatarsal heads (ball of the foot), while at the same time maintaining balance for as long as possible with the heel lifted off the ground for up to five seconds as in figure 7.8 and so on until the end of the course.
4 The subject continues to the end mark and the score is calculated (see analysis).

Analysis

Although normative data for this particular test is uncommon, a scoring system can be used to provide baseline information for subsequent testing as shown in table 7.5.

Fig. 7.7 Set-up for the bass dynamic test

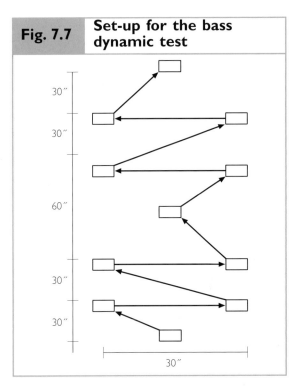

Fig. 7.8 A subject undergoing a bass dynamic test

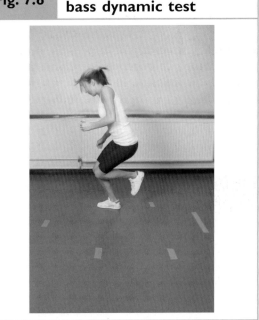

Table 7.5	Scoring sheet for bass dynamic test	
Points added		**Points scored**
5 points	Successfully covering the landing mark with the foot.	
1 point	For each second the subject remains balanced (up to 5 sec).	
A total of 10 points is possible for each mark, with a perfect score being 100 points.		
Points deducted		
-5 points	Failing to stop on landing on a given hop (i.e. taking more hops).	
-5 points	Failing to completely cover the mark.	
-5 points	If any other body part touches the floor on landing.	
-1 point	For each second the foot moves while in the balance position.	
	Total points =	

Agility testing

Several tests can be used as a measure of agility; however, most of these only measure change of direction speed (and therefore should be called change of direction tests), as most sports involve reacting to random stimuli within a game situation.

For the purpose of this book, all the following tests will be referred to as agility tests. As with the sprint tests, a stopwatch can be used but light gates would be much more accurate. Also, try to test on a surface that is the same as the one used for the sport.

Two of the most common agility tests are the *Illinois agility test* as set out in figure 7.9 and the *t-test* as shown in figure 7.10.

Illinois agility test

Although some research states that the Illinois agility test is possibly less valid than other agility tests, it is easy to administer and requires little in the way of resources. The test is used quite extensively in all types of sport.

Required resources

Flat surface, tape measure, eight cones, stopwatch (or light gates).

Set-up

The length of the course is 10 metres and the width (distance between the start and finish points) is 5 metres. Four cones are used to mark the start, finish, and the two turning points. The cones in the centre are spaced 3.3 metres apart as can be seen in figure 7.9.

Testing method

1. The subject lies face down on the floor (indoors or outdoors) at the start point of the course, behind the line and facing the direction of the course.
2. On the tester's command, the subject jumps to their feet and negotiates the course around the cones to the finish point as quickly as possible.
3. The tester should record the total time taken to complete the agility course.
4. The subject must ensure that they go around the cones and not step on any, as this will result in that particular test run being cancelled.
5. The test can be repeated as many times as possible, but rest periods should be given between attempts.
6. If repeated tests become slower, this is usually an indication that the subject is becoming fatigued. If this is the case, the test should be postponed to another day.

Analysis

Analysis of the Illinois agility test results can be done by comparing them with the results of previous tests and using them as a motivation for future improvement. Team sports often publish results as a motivational tool for team members.

Classification

The published classifications for agility testing for adults (male and female) and 16-year-olds can be found in tables 7.6a and 7.6b.

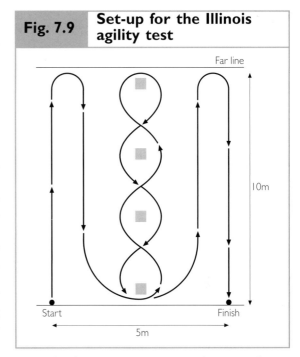

Fig. 7.9 Set-up for the Illinois agility test

Far line

10m

Start

Finish

5m

Note: If subsequent testing is to be carried out, you must ensure that the test is performed on the same surface in order to increase the repeatability of the test. It is also important when starting the test to record the time from the point at which the starter gives the command, and not the point at which the subject crosses the start line.

Table 7.6a	Normative Illinois agility data for adults (values-in-seconds)				
Gender	Excellent	Above average	Average	Below average	Poor
Male	<15.2	15.2–16.1	16.2–18.1	18.2–19.3	>19.3
Female	<17.0	17.0–17.9	18.0–21.7	21.8–23.0	>23.0

Table 7.6b	Normative Illinois agility data for 16-year-olds (values-in-seconds)				
Gender	Excellent	Above average	Average	Below average	Poor
Male	<15.9	15.9–16.7	16.8–17.6	17.7–18.8	>18.8
Female	<17.5	17.5–18.6	18.7–22.4	22.5–23.4	>23.4

T-test

Required resources

Flat surface, tape measure, four cones, stopwatch (or light gates).

Set-up

The length and width of the course is 10 yards and the width (distance between the start and finish points) is five yards. Four cones are used to mark the start, finish and the two turning points. Each turning cone is spaced five metres from the centre line as can be seen in figure 7.9. Subjects should be careful not to cross their feet when shuffling.

Testing method

1. The subject sprints from the start cone on the tester's command (start stopwatch) to touch the centre cone with their hand.
2. The subject then shuffles side-step to touch the left cone with the left hand.
3. The subject then shuffles side-step to touch the right cone with the right hand.
4. The subject then shuffles side-step to touch

Fig. 7.10   Set-up for the t-test

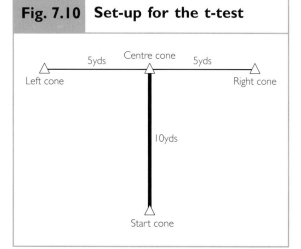

Table 7.7	T-test classification for adult team sports	
	Male (sec)	Female (sec)
Excellent	<9.5	<10.5
Good	9.6 to 10.5	10.6 to 11.5
Average	10.6 to 11.5	11.6 to 12.5
Poor	>11.6	>12.6

the centre cone, then runs backwards past the start cone.

5. The time is measured as the subject passes the start cone.

505 agility test

The t-test can be modified and made more sport or skill specific. For example, field hockey or basketball players could perform the test while controlling the ball. The 505 agility test is one such adapted test.

The 505 agility test is an assessment of a subject's ability to change direction and correlates well with their acceleration. Subjects sprint towards a cone 15 metres away. Timing starts when they pass through timing gates (or by use of a stopwatch) at 10 metres. The time it takes to run a further five metres, turn around 180°, and run back to the timing gates (or finish) is recorded. The distance covered is 10 metres, with one change of direction.

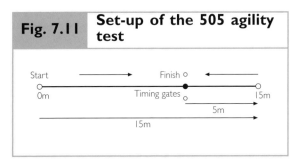

Fig. 7.11	Set-up of the 505 agility test

Balsom run

The Balsom run is an agility test developed by Paul Balsom in 1994. It requires a few practice runs to familiarise subjects with the route. Players have to perform several changes in direction and two turns in this test. The total time to complete the run is 11.7 seconds in a sample of elite English Premier League soccer players.

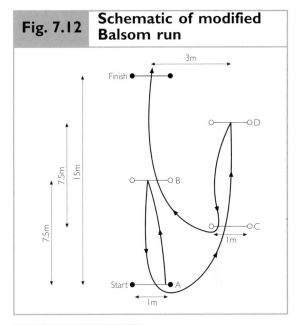

Fig. 7.12	Schematic of modified Balsom run

Required resources

Flat surface, tape measure, cones, stopwatch (or light gates).

Set-up

The length of the course is 15 metres. Cones are used to mark the start, finish and the three turning points as shown in figure 7.12.

Testing method

1. The subject starts at A and runs to cones at B before turning and returning to A.
2. Subject runs through cones at C, turns back at D, and returns through C.
3. Subject turns to the right and runs through cones at B and through the finish.
4. Total time is recorded.

Further reading

Atwater, A. E. (1979) 'Kinematic analysis of striding during the sprint start and mid-race sprint'. *Medicine and Science in Sports and Exercise*, 11: p. 85

Balsom, P. (1994) 'Evaluation of physical performance'. In Ekblom, B. (ed.) *Football (soccer)*, Oxford, UK: Blackwell Scientific, p. 112

Barnes, C. (2007) 'Soccer'. In Winter, E. M., Jones, A. M., Davison, R. C., Bromley, P. & Mercer, T. (eds.) *Sport and Exercise Science Testing Guidelines: The British Association of Sport and Exercise Sciences Guide. Volume I: Sport Testing*, London and New York: Routledge, pp. 241-8

Barrow, H. & McGee, R. (1971) *A Practical Approach to Measurement in Physical Education*, Philadelphia, Pennsylvania: Lea & Febiger

Baumgartner, T. & Jackson, A. (1975) *Measurement for Evaluation in Physical Education*, Boston, Massachusetts: Houghton Mifflin

Blazevich, T. (1997a) 'Resistance training for sprinters (part 1): Theoretical considerations'. *Strength and Conditioning Coach*, 4: pp. 9-12

Blazevich, T. (1997b) 'Resistance training for sprinters (part 2): Exercise suggestions'. *Strength and Conditioning Coach*, 5: pp. 5-10

Bloomfield, J., Ackland, T. R. & Elliot, B. C. (1994) *Applied Anatomy and Biomechanics in Sport*, Melbourne, Australia: Blackwell Scientific

Booher, L. D., Hench, K. M., Worrell, T. W. & Stikeleather, J. (1993) 'Reliability of three single-leg hops tests'. *Journal of Sport Rehabilitation*, 2: pp. 165-70

Burggemann, G. & Glad, B. (Glad, B. ed.) (1990) 'Time analysis of the sprint events. Scientific Research Project at the Games of the XXIVth Olympiad-Seoul 1988'. International Athletic Foundation, Monaco. pp. 11-89

Buttifant, D., Graham, K. & Cross, K. (1999) 'Agility and speed in soccer players are two different performance parameters'. Paper presented at the Science and Football IV Conference, Sydney, NSW

Chelladurai, P., Yuhasz, M. & Sipura, R. (1977) 'The reactive agility test'. *Perceptual and Motor Skills*, 44: pp. 1319-24

Clark, S., Martin, D., Lee, H., Fornasiero, D. & Quinn, A. (1998) 'Relationship between speed and agility in nationally ranked junior tennis players'. Paper presented at the Australian Conference of Science and Medicine in Sport 1998, Adelaide, SA

Colby, S., Francisco, A., Yu, B., Kirkendall, D., Finch, M. & Garrett, W. (2000) 'Electromyographic and kinematic analysis of cutting manoeuvres'. *American Journal of Sports Medicine*, 28: pp. 234-40

Delecluse, C. (1997) 'Influence of strength training on sprint running performance'. *Sports Medicine*, 24: pp. 148-56

Delecluse, C., Van Coppennolle, H., Willem, E., Van Leemputte, M., Diels, R. & Goris, M. (1995) 'Influence of high-resistance and high-velocity training on sprint performance'. *Medicine and Science in Sports and Exercise*, 27: pp. 1203-9

Djevalikian, R. (1993) 'The relationship between asymmetrical leg power and change of running direction'. University of North Carolina, Chapel Hill, NC – unpublished master's thesis

Donati, A. (1996) 'The association between the development of strength and speed'. *New Studies in Athletics*, 2: pp. 51-8

Draper, J. A. & Lancaster, M. G. (1985) 'The 505 test: A test for agility in the horizontal plane'. *Australian Journal of Science and Medicine in Sport*, 17: pp. 15-18

Gore, C. J. (2000) 'Physiological tests for elite athletes'. Australian Sports Commission. Canberra, ACT

Hastad, D. N. & Lacy, A. C. (1994) *Measurement and Evaluation in Physical Education and Exercise Science*, 2nd edn, Scottsdale, Arizona: Gorsuch Scarisbrick

Hertel, J., Denegar, C. R., Johnson, P. D., Hale, S. A. & Buckely, W. E. (1999) 'Reliability of the cybex reactor in the assessment of an agility task'. *Journal of Sport Rehabilitation*, 8: pp. 24-31

Hoffman, K. (1971) 'Stature, leg length and stride frequency'. *Track Technique*, 46: pp. 1463-9

Johnson, B. L. & Nelson, J. K. (1969) *Practical measurements for evaluation in physical education*, Minneapolis, Minnesota: Burgess

Kukolj, M., Ropret, R., Ugarkovic, D. & Jaric, S. (1999) 'Anthropometric, strength, and power predictors of sprinting performance'. *Journal of Sports Medicine and Physical Fitness*, 39: pp. 120-2

Kyrolainen, H., Komi, P. & Belli, A. (1999) 'Changes in muscle activity patterns and kinetics with increasing running speed'. *Journal of Strength and Conditioning Research*, 13: pp. 400-6

Mann, R. V. (1981) 'A kinetic analysis of sprinting'. *Medicine and Science in Sports and Exercise*, 13: pp. 325-8

McCurdy, K. & Lanford, G. (2006) 'The relationship between maximum unilateral squat strength and balance in young adult men and women'. *Journal of Sports Science and Medicine*, 5: pp. 282-8

Pauole, K., Madole, K., Garhammer, J., Lacourse, M. & Rozenek, R. (2000) 'Reliability and validity of the t-test as a measure of agility, leg power, and leg speed in college-aged men and women'. *Journal of Strength and Conditioning Research*, 14: pp. 443-50

Psotta, R., & Bunc, V. (2003) 'Intermittent anaerobic running test (IAnRT) reliability and factor validity in soccer players'. *Communication to the Fifth World Congress of Science and Football*, Madrid, Spain: Editorial Gymnos, p. 94

Rompottie, K. (1972). 'A study of stride length in running'. *International Track and Field*, pp. 249-56

Roozen, M. (2004) 'Illinois agility test'. *NSCA's Performance Training Journal*, 3: pp. 5-6

Sheppard, J. (2003) 'Strength and conditioning exercise selection in speed development'. *Strength and Conditioning Journal*, 25: pp. 26-30

Sheppard, J. (2004) 'Improving the sprint start with strength and conditioning exercise'. *Modern Athlete and Coach*, 42: pp. 9-13

Young, W. B., Benton, D., Duthie, G. & Pryor, J. (2001) 'Resistance training for short sprints and maximum-speed sprints'. *Strength and Conditioning Journal*, 23: pp. 7-13

Young, W. B., James, R. & Montgomery, I. (2002) 'Is muscle power related to running speed with changes of direction?' *Journal of Sports Medicine and Physical Fitness*, 43: pp. 282-8

Young, W. B., McLean, B. & Ardagna, J. (1995) 'Relationship between strength qualities and sprinting performance'. *Journal of Sports Medicine and Physical Fitness*, 35: pp. 13-19

POWER TESTING

OBJECTIVES

After completing this chapter you should be able to:

1 Explain the term 'power' in the context of cardiovascular- and resistance-type exercises.

2 Explain the difference between the terms 'anaerobic capacity' and 'anaerobic power'.

3 Discuss how jumping ability is considered to be important in terms of testing for power.

4 Discuss the origin of jump testing and how it has developed over the years.

5 Explain the relationship between power, force and velocity in skeletal muscle.

6 Apply various methods of converting jump height during testing into a measurement of power.

7 Understand the stretch-shortening cycle utilised in jumping.

8 Explain the concept of oxygen debt and how it can be used to estimate anaerobic power.

9 Discuss the various field and laboratory tests that can be used to determine power.

10 Understand the concept of 'critical power' and how it can be used to predict performance in high-intensity and endurance sports.

Power

As you may remember, the term 'power' was defined in chapter 2 in relation to cardiovascular and resistance exercises, and it was noted that

the anaerobic system was an important means of testing power.

The anaerobic system can be thought of as consisting of two main components, *anaerobic power* and *anaerobic capacity* (see figure 8.1). Anaerobic power is often described as *'the maximal rate of anaerobic energy production during exercise'*, whereas anaerobic capacity can be described as *'the total amount of energy that can be produced anaerobically during exercise'*.

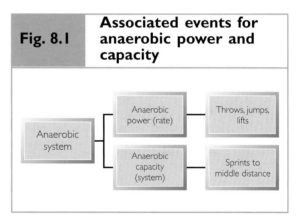

Fig. 8.1 Associated events for anaerobic power and capacity

Testing for power

Anaerobic capacity is important for events such as sprinting and middle distance running, whereas anaerobic power is considered to be important for throwing and jumping events.

The standing vertical jump has been used extensively as one of the most common tests to evaluate power of the lower limbs, as it represents the *jumping ability* that is a common requirement in many different sports.

One of the many methods for testing vertical jump is by using an electrical, pressure sensitive jump mat. This measures the length of time the subject is in the air when jumping, and from this information it can calculate the height of the jump (some devices will calculate this whereas others require the tester to calculate the jump height). A device known as a *force plate* can also calculate the flight time of an individual to a high degree of accuracy.

Another method widely used is to mark a board with chalk as high as possible while performing a vertical jump; however, this is much less accurate than some of the other methods.

There are many other tests for assessing muscular power, which include the standing broad jump or long jump.

The origin of vertical jump testing

The original *vertical jump test* was one of the first tests ever to be developed to investigate muscular power. A researcher called Sargent developed and described the test methodology in 1921 and it is still often referred to as the *Sargent jump*.

One of the main reasons for performing vertical jump testing is that it reflects the strength capabilities of the knee and hip extensor muscles; however, due to the nature of the technique during performance, the test can also be affected (both negatively and positively) by certain factors, which must be kept consistent during all tests. Three of the main factors that can affect the outcome of the test are:

• Arm swing
• Countermovement
• Knee angle at start position

Including an arm swing during the jump increases the skill level and can also positively affect the vertical jump height achieved. In order to standardise tests, some forms of testing protocol require subjects to jump with their hands on their hips. Other test protocols allow free arm-movement.

A *countermovement jump* is where the subject performs a short initial descent followed by an explosive jump (this is sometimes known as a pre-stretch). If the jump is performed without a pre-stretch from a stationary semi-squatted position, this is known as a *squat jump*.

The pre-stretch can have a considerable effect on the jump outcome. For instance, an average individual with a countermovement jump height of 40cm would typically achieve a squat jump of nearer 34–36cm (more than 10 per cent difference in some cases). The main reason for this difference in outcome is that the lack of a countermovement results in no pre-stretching of the muscles and tendons. There is therefore no use of the stretch shortening cycle or elastic potential, which is responsible for much of the force production in vertical jumping (Coulson and Archer 2008).

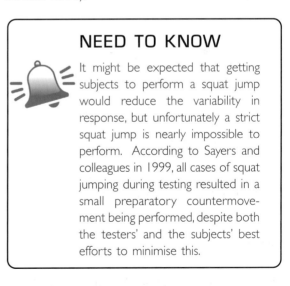

NEED TO KNOW

It might be expected that getting subjects to perform a squat jump would reduce the variability in response, but unfortunately a strict squat jump is nearly impossible to perform. According to Sayers and colleagues in 1999, all cases of squat jumping during testing resulted in a small preparatory countermovement being performed, despite both the testers' and the subjects' best efforts to minimise this.

One-legged vertical jump testing

Many athletes possess a good two-legged vertical jump, but a poor one-legged jump, particularly on their non-dominant side. In sports such as basketball or soccer, most jumping is from one leg.

The protocol of one-legged testing is much more demanding than two-legged testing, and subjects must be reasonably strong and familiar with the movement. One-legged testing is best performed on a force plate. Subjects should have the contralateral leg bent at 90° and arms crossed over the chest. A countermovement can be performed but the knee angle should not exceed 90°. The measurement obtained from the force plate is ground reaction force and should be expressed as a percentage of the subject's bodyweight. Typical values should be approximately 2 per cent of the bodyweight of the subject being tested.

Jump and reach test

This jump test is simple to administer and relatively inexpensive as there are minimal resources required.

One of the limitations of testing using a wall is that it may impede jumping technique and hence result in lower measures of vertical jump height (Canavan and Vescovi 2004). An individual's shoulder flexibility and trunk bending can also affect the values obtained.

Required resources

A wall, one-metre tape measure, chalk.

Testing method

1. The subject chalks the end of the fingertips.
2. The subject then stands side-on to the wall, keeping both feet on the ground and reaches up as high as possible with one hand to mark the wall with the tips of the fingers (mark 1).

Fig. 8.2	**(a) Mark 1 – vertical jump test**	**(b) Mark 2 – vertical jump test**

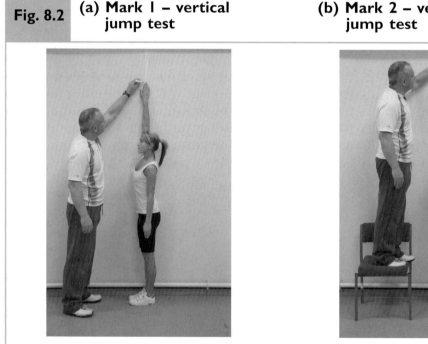
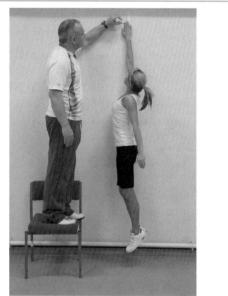

3. From a static position, the subject jumps as high as possible and marks the wall with the chalk on the fingertips (mark 2).
4. The depth of jump should be around 90° knee flexion, depending on the subject's strength.
5. The tester then measures the distance from mark 1 to mark 2. The test can be performed as many times as the subject wishes.

Analysis

Scores from the vertical jump tests should be recorded and used as a baseline measurement to compare against subsequent test scores in order to monitor improvement.

Jump-belts

One way to overcome the problems associated with wall jump testing is to use a jump-belt. The subject securely attaches a belt around their waist, to which a wire from a mat on the ground is attached. The displacement of the wire from a normal standing position (having ensured that the instrument is zeroed beforehand) is the vertical jump height in centimetres. One aspect often neglected is that the subject should land with almost straight legs; landing with bent legs increases jump time and hence overestimates vertical jump height.

Although easy to administer in terms of methodology, this type of test (also referred to as a squat jump test) can be relatively expensive to carry out, depending on the type of resources used and the environment in which testing takes place.

Required resources

Jump-belt.

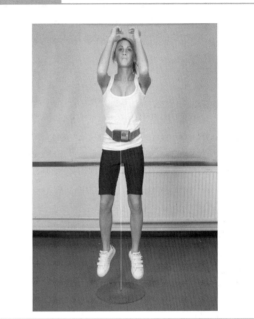

Fig. 8.3 Testing using a jump-belt

Testing method

1. The subject should attach the jump-belt around the waist.
2. The subject either bends the knees to 90°, stands still for one second and then jumps as high as possible without performing a countermovement, or jumps using a countermovement, depending on the protocol (figure 8.3).
3. The subject should land with straight legs and the vertical jump height measured on the device.
4. The test should be repeated several times without fatigue to the subject.

Analysis

As with previous jump tests, scores should be recorded and used to compare against subsequent test scores in order to monitor improvement.

Jump timing mats

Squat jump testing can also be performed more accurately by using specialised equipment such as timing mats. With this equipment, the vertical jump is calculated by the duration of time in the air.

The jump mat contains electronic contacts, which are broken when the subject is not touching the mat, and are re-formed when the subject returns to the mat.

Vertical jump measurements are often highest using timing mats due to a slight change in the subject's centre of gravity (on average 4–5cm).

Required resources

Jump timing mat.

Testing method

1. The subject should stand in the middle of the timing mat.
2. The subject bends the knees to 90°, stands still for one second and jumps as high as possible without performing a countermovement, or jumps using a countermovement, depending on the protocol.
3. The subject should land with straight legs and the flight time read from the device. The centre of gravity must return to the same position on landing as on take-off.
4. The test should be repeated several times without fatigue to the subject.

Analysis

The following equation (proposed by Bosco in 1983) can be used to calculate jump height:

Height (cm) = [(time in air)^2 × g/8] × 100

[time in air]^2 × 1.226 × 100
where g = acceleration due to gravity
= 9.81m.s^{-2}

| Fig. 8.4 | Jump timing mat testing |

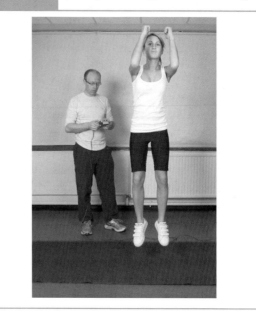

Force platforms

A force platform is frequently used in biomechanics. It produces voltage signals proportional to the forces applied to the surface of the platform in different directions.

Vertical jump can be estimated using different techniques with a force platform: these are (1) flight time, (2) impulse momentum theory and (3) work-energy theory. The simplest of these is the flight-time technique. By measuring ground reaction force, the time taken between take-off and landing can be estimated, and then vertical jump height can be calculated from the previous equation.

Required resources

Force platform, calculator.

Testing method

1. The subject should stand in the middle of the force platform.
2. The subject either bends the knees to 90°, stands still for one second and then jumps as high as possible without performing a countermovement, or jumps using a countermovement, depending on the protocol.
3. The subject should land with straight legs and the flight time read from the device. The centre of gravity must return to the same position on landing as on take-off.
4. The test should be repeated several times without fatigue to the subject.

Analysis

As for jump timing mat testing, the Bosco equation can be used to calculate jump height:

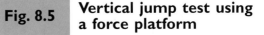

$$\text{Height (cm)} = [(\text{time in air})^2 \times g/8] \times 100$$

$$[\text{time in air}]^2 \times 1.226 \times 100$$

where g = acceleration due to gravity = $9.81\,\text{m.s}^{-2}$

Fig. 8.5	Vertical jump test using a force platform

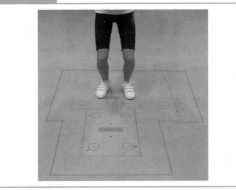

Classification

Table 8.1a	Normative data for adults (cm) for the vertical jump	
Rating	Male	Female
Excellent	>65	>58
Good	50–65	47–58
Average	40–49	36–46
Fair	30–39	26–35
Poor	<30	<26

Table 8.1b	Normative data for the vertical jump for 15 to 16-year-olds (cm)				
Gender	Excellent	Good	Average	Fair	Poor
Male	>65	56–65	50–55	40–49	<40
Female	>60	51–60	41–50	35–40	<35

Calculating power

It is useful to express the results of vertical jump testing in units of power. One of the older methods used is the equation proposed by Lewis in 1981:

Predicted average power (Watts) =

$21.72 \times$ subject mass (kg) $\times$ square root of the jump height (m)

The accuracy of the Lewis equation has been called into question by authors such as Canavan and Vescovi in 2004 who suggested that the power prediction equation of Harman et al. (1991) is a more accurate method for conversion. The equation proposed by Harman et al. is:

Predicted average power (Watts) =

$23.0 \times$ subject mass (kg) $+ 21.2 \times$ jump height (cm) $- 1393$

NEED TO KNOW

When expressed as power divided by body mass or W/kg, vertical jump measurements for males range from 15.8 W/kg for regional athletes and 16.7 W/kg for national level athletes and 17.4 W/kg for international athletes. For females, the respective values are 13.6, 14.4 and 15.7 W/kg (Logan et al. 2000) – calculated using the Lewis equation.

Tests of vertical jump height for male British national league basketball players resulted in values of 24–59cm with an average of 47cm. For their female equivalents, tests resulted in values of 21–41cm with an average of 33cm (Harley and Doust 1997).

Note: These values are lower than those obtained in elite professional basketball players competing in leagues such as the NBA.

Power measurement using transducers

Forces can be developed by the human body in different planes and axes such as the sagittal, transverse and frontal. Some of these movements are linear and some are rotational (or angular), and can be a combination of all planes in one movement.

A simple example of different plane movement is that of a jab or a hook in boxing. A jab that is a short, sharp punching movement in the transverse plane is predominantly linear in nature whereas a hook is more of a rotational movement, which combines both the transverse and frontal planes.

A linear transducer (the term given to a device that changes one form of energy to another) produces an electrical signal which is proportional to any movement that is carried out (by the structure to which it is attached). This movement (or displacement) is typically recorded as a voltage and it is this voltage signal, that is amplified and filtered through a device and then converted into digital information via a computer interface. This converted data is then compared to calibration values, which have been developed as a result of years of testing by the manufacturer.

Much important and relevant data can be obtained from linear transducers including:

- Power
- Force
- Velocity
- Acceleration
- Displacement

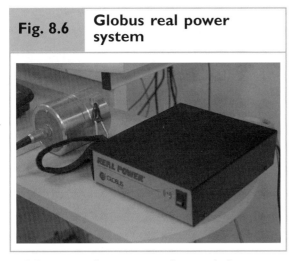

Fig. 8.6 Globus real power system

Most transducers manufactured for testing movement within a limited space comprise a cable connected to a PC interface.

Figure 8.6 shows a Globus real power transducer system, which the authors use regularly.

For operational purposes, the cable connected to the transducer can be attached to the subject or an object that the subject is moving.

The transducer system can be used to measure a large range of sport- or event-specific movements. Punch and kick forces and power can be measured when the cable is connected to the wrist or ankle.

Figure 8.7 shows how kicking in sports such as martial arts or soccer can be tested using the transducer system. Figure 8.8 shows how punching in sports such as boxing can be tested.

The cable is also often attached to a barbell or dumbbell, but can be used with a variety of objects such as the shot in shot-putting.

Using the manufacturer's software, the mass of the object to be moved is input, for example an 80kg barbell. The device then monitors the displacement (distance the bar moved), speed and acceleration of the object 100 times per

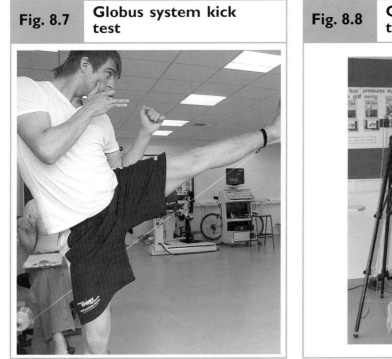

Fig. 8.7 Globus system kick test

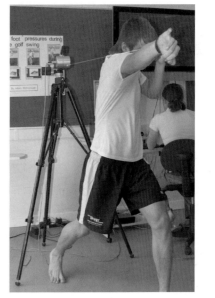

Fig. 8.8 Globus system punch test

Table 8.2	Peak force and power scores for punching and kicking before and after a 10-week training camp			
	Front leg front kick	Back leg front kick	Punch (left jab)	Punch (right cross)
Month	Peak Force Peak Power	Peak Force Peak Power	Peak Force Peak Power	Peak Force Peak Power
Jan	860N 5400W	960N 5400W	270N 1540W	290N 1800W
March	1000N 5900W	1150N 7000W	290N 1640W	300N 1950W

second. It can then calculate the power, force and velocity throughout the movement every 10 milliseconds, producing an output trace.

There is a lack of normative data for punching and kicking power; however, we have the data shown in figure 8.8 from a professional kickboxer for punch and kick force, power and velocity. Through repeated testing, you may develop your own normative data.

There is a wide variety of different exercises/movements that a linear encoder can be used for, and one of its greatest benefits is how directly relevant it can be to sports-specific movements.

Standing broad jump

Standing broad jumps are often performed in specific sports such as long-jumping or triple jumping as a more specific measure of lower body strength.

The standing broad-jump test is also frequently performed as a test of local muscular performance for children because it is simple to perform and can be administered with minimal equipment for large groups.

Required resources

Long-jump pit or appropriate jump area, 30-metre tape measure.

Testing method

1. The subject places their feet on the start line of the designated jump area.
2. The start of the jump must be performed from a static position.
3. The subject crouches, leans forward, swings their arms backwards, and then jumps horizontally as far as possible, taking off with both feet simultaneously.
4. The tester should measure from the start line to the nearest point of contact on the jump area surface.
5. Subjects can have several attempts and the greatest distance achieved is recorded.

Analysis

All subjects' scores from this test should be recorded and used as a baseline measurement to compare against subsequent test scores in order to monitor improvement.

Classification

It is difficult to have a general 'one-fits-all' classification table for this test as there are many variables that can affect the outcome of the test, such as age, gender and experience.

One of the main variables that could also

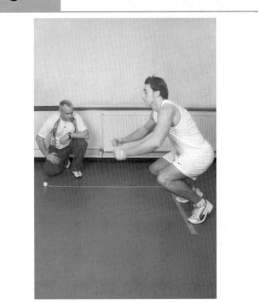

Fig. 8.9 **Standing broad jump**

affect the outcome of the test is the surface of the designated jump area with respect to take-off and landing. A firmer take-off surface would allow the subject to gain more purchase than a softer take-off surface, and having a sandpit would probably encourage a greater jump because of the softer landing.

The general environment could also affect the outcome, as jumping into a headwind would obviously reduce the potential of the jump.

The age, gender and background status of the subject are the main factors in determining the outcome of the jump, so take these into consideration when trying to determine the classification of each subject after any testing has taken place. Although there are many classification tables relevant to different subject groups, table 8.3a provides a ranking for world-class athletes (shown in percentage terms), whereas table 8.3b gives a classification for younger individuals (shown in performance-rating terms).

Table 8.3a	Data for broad jump obtained from world-class athletes (values-in-metres)	
% Rank	Female	Male
91–100	2.94–3.15	3.40–3.75
81–90	2.80–2.93	3.10–3.39
71–80	2.65–2.79	2.95–3.09
61–70	2.50–2.64	2.80–2.94
51–60	2.35–2.49	2.65–2.79
41–50	2.20–2.34	2.50–2.64
31–40	2.05–2.19	2.35–2.49
21–30	1.90–2.04	2.20–2.34
11–20	1.75–1.89	2.05–2.19
1–10	1.60–1.74	1.90–2.04

Table 8.3b	Normative data for broad jump for 15 to 16-year-olds (values-in-metres)				
Gender	Excellent	Above Average	Average	Below Average	Poor
Male	>2.00	2.00–1.86	1.85–1.76	1.75–1.65	<1.65
Female	>1.65	1.65–1.56	1.55–1.46	1.45–1.35	<1.35

Anaerobic capacity

Anaerobic capacity, which was defined earlier (see page 166), can also be described as 'the total amount of energy that can be produced anaerobically during exercise'. While determination, or measurement, of aerobic capacity (otherwise known as VO_2 max) is a relatively simple process as described in chapter 9, unfortunately this is not the case for anaerobic capacity (or the total amount of energy produced anaerobically during exercise). This type of measurement is usually restricted to laboratory environments. Two of the most common measurement methods, which can be used to estimate the anaerobic energy produced, are known as 'excess post-exercise oxygen consumption' and 'maximal accumulated oxygen deficit'.

Excess post-exercise oxygen consumption (EPOC)

The seemingly long-winded term 'excess post-exercise oxygen consumption' refers to the increase in oxygen consumption above rest. It occurs after a bout of exercise in order to replenish the ATP and PCr stores used. EPOC is also used to facilitate the breakdown of any lactate produced during a bout of high-intensity exercise for conversion to provide a further energy source of ATP.

The degree of the anaerobic contribution to the bout of high-intensity exercise can be estimated by measuring the excess post-exercise oxygen consumption (this was formerly termed the *oxygen debt*). This method, however, is not currently in common use as it has generally been superceded by a more accurate method known as *maximal accumulated oxygen deficit,* also used as a measurement of anaerobic capacity.

Maximal accumulated oxygen deficit (MAOD)

For this more current method of testing anaerobic capacity, the relationship between an individual's oxygen uptake (VO_2) and power during sub-maximal exercise is measured (usually by means of a treadmill or cycle ergometer). This relationship is then used to provide (using a specific calculation) a reasonably accurate estimate of the oxygen requirements of the exercise performed (fig. 8.10).

The difference between the amount of oxygen consumed during the exercise bout and the estimated oxygen requirement for that bout is termed the *oxygen deficit*. The oxygen deficit obtained by an individual during exhaustive maximal exercise of between 2 and 3 minutes is termed the *maximal accumulated oxygen deficit*.

This type of testing is usually carried out by

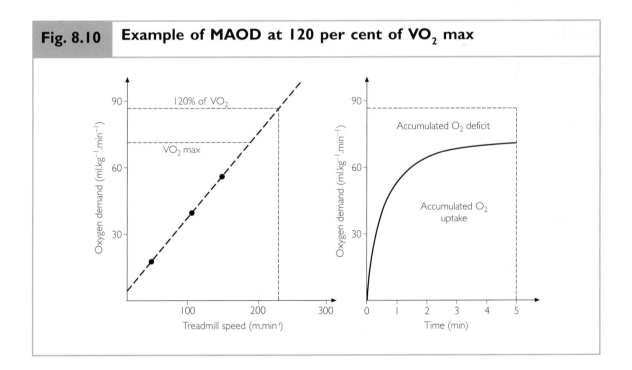

Fig. 8.10 **Example of MAOD at 120 per cent of VO₂ max**

experienced testers under laboratory conditions, although it can be done in a field environment if portable testing equipment is available. Research has shown that exercises of 2–5 minutes usually produce the greatest value of maximal accumulated oxygen deficit.

According to research, the principle of testing for maximal accumulated oxygen deficit is to estimate the oxygen requirements (during a particular bout of exercise performed above VO_2 max), and then measure the actual oxygen consumption during the same bout of exercise.

Some of the limitations related to the measurement of MAOD are the requirement for gas analysis, which can be expensive and time consuming for subjects to be highly motivated to work to exhaustion at very high intensity levels. Also, this method only estimates the oxygen requirements for the subject and there is large potential for error in this estimation.

Advantages of MAOD testing as a measure of anaerobic capacity are that it isolates the anaerobic contribution and has been supported by biochemical measurements.

When performing these tests, an intensity of approximately 120 per cent of VO_2 max is estimated and oxygen consumption (VO_2) is calculated. Values of maximal accumulated oxygen deficit can vary from 2.8 litres in females to 7.5 litres in sprint-trained males.

Cunningham-Faulkner anaerobic test

This simple, laboratory-based method of estimating an individual's anaerobic performance capacity was developed in Australia in 1969. For many sports, such as soccer, rugby and hockey, the running in the test is considered to be a more relevant form of exercise testing than using a cycle ergometer. The test is simply administered by measuring the time to exhaustion at 12.9 km.h^{-1} at a 20 per cent gradient.

Required resources

Treadmill with capacity to increase gradient rapidly to 20 per cent, stopwatch, HR monitor and blood lactate analyser (optional).

Testing method

1. Ensure the treadmill is set at 0 per cent incline.
2. The subject warms up for 6 minutes at 8km.h^{-1}, followed by 2 minutes at 12.9kmh.$^{-1}$, and finishing with a further 2 minutes at 3.5km.h^{-1}.
3. Subject should have a brief break and stretch.
4. Set the treadmill to 12.9km.h^{-1} (8mph) and an incline of 20 per cent.
5. Start timing when the athlete can run unsupported, and finish when they grip the handrail.
6. Subjects need to be strongly encouraged during the test, as they must work to exhaustion, running up a steep slope.
7. Have crash mats and a spotter in a safe position behind the treadmill in the unlikely event that the subject should fall off the treadmill.
8. Record length of sprint to nearest 0.5 seconds, and monitor peak heart rate.
9. Post-exercise blood lactate concentration could be measured at 4 minutes post-test as an indicator of anaerobic metabolism.

Analysis

Scores should be recorded and used to compare against subsequent test scores in order to monitor improvement.

Classification

Table 8.4 (overleaf) provides typical times to exhaustion recorded when testing sample groups of regional, national and international games players.

Table 8.4	Normative data for the Cunningham-Faulkner Test	
Regional games players (sec)	National games players (sec)	International games players (sec)
54.4 ± 8.8	66.2 ± 10.7	80.6 ± 12.0

Wingate anaerobic cycle test (WAnT)

The Wingate anaerobic 30 cycle test was developed during the 1970s at the Wingate Institute in Israel. It has been one of the most popular anaerobic tests to date, but as a cycle-ergometer test it is more specific to cycle-based sports.

NEED TO KNOW

Being very convenient, cycle ergometers are frequently used to measure anaerobic power output, anaerobic capacity and fatigue.

The WAnT can be used to assess power in a wide variety of populations from young people with disabilities to highly trained track cyclists. The exercise is performed maximally and the most commonly used test duration is 30 seconds. Pedal frequencies can reach 170rpm in the first few seconds, falling to nearer 80rpm towards the end of the 30-second period.

As outlined in chapter 2, a 30-second Wingate test would be primarily anaerobic (80 per cent anaerobic). For the lesser used, 5-second Wingate test, the anaerobic contribution would be even greater (92 per cent anaerobic).

The original Wingate test was developed using a standardised load of 0.075kg per kg of the subject's body mass. For example, for a 70kg person the flywheel resistance should be 5.25kg (70kg × 0.075). However, Oded Bar-Or (a much published researcher in this field), in his review of the Wingate test in 1987, recommended the use of 0.090kg/kg body mass for adult non-athletes and 0.100kg/kg body mass in adult athletes. So, for the example of the 70kg adult athlete, the load applied to maximise peak power should be 7kg (70kg × 0.1).

Full details on how to administer the Wingate test can be obtained from the book written by Inbar, Bar-Or and Skinner in 1996.

Wingate testing can be performed on a standard Monark ergometer fitted with a photocell or mechanical counter that records rpm at either 1 or 5 second intervals. The use of electro-mechanically-braked cycle ergometers such as the Lode allows recording at one-second intervals.

There is significant inertia (resistance to movement) of the flywheel when using friction-braked ergometers such as the Monark. Because of this, the initial high rpm produced before the load is applied means that a significant amount of energy has already been accumulated before the 30-second test, resulting in over-estimates of peak and average power. When using Monark ergometers this inertia should be accounted for in calculations.

A recent study in 2006 by the researchers Micklewright and colleagues from the University of Essex in the UK demonstrated that Wingate testing performed on both mechanically-braked (Monark) and electromechanically-braked (Lode) cycle ergometers, while producing valid measures of anaerobic fitness, also produced markedly different values from each other. So, quite surprisingly, values from a Wingate test on a Monark ergometer are not directly comparable to those obtained from a Lode ergometer, due to differing test protocols and the inertia issue.

A similar test to the Wingate has also been devised called the Quebec 10-second test, which attempts to overcome the problem of inertia, but it remains much less commonly used than the standard Wingate test.

Required resources

Cycle ergometer, stopwatch.

Testing method

1. The subject performs a 5-minute standardised warm-up on the ergometer at 60 or 100W.
2. The subject then begins pedalling as fast as possible without any resistance. Within 3 seconds, a fixed resistance is applied to the flywheel and the subject continues to pedal 'all out' for 30 seconds.
3. This resistance is applied automatically using an electromechanically-braked ergometer, or manually when using a Monark cycle ergometer.
4. Subjects should be encouraged to fight fatigue and cycle maximally throughout the 30 seconds.

Note: The difference between the Monark and Lode protocols is that the subject is allowed 3 seconds before the braking force is applied when using a Monark, whereas this force is applied instantaneously in the case of the Lode.

Fig. 8.12 **The Wingate anaerobic cycle test**

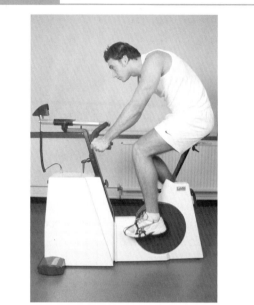

Analysis

There are several parameters that can be measured as a result of performing this particular test. The most common are:

1. Peak power output
2. Relative peak power output
3. Anaerobic capacity
4. Fatigue index

1. Peak power output (PP)

Peak power output is the greatest output over a 5-second period. This is usually reached in the first 2–3 seconds of testing. The following equation can be used to calculate peak power output with a Monark ergometer:

Peak power output = (flywheel rpm for highest 5s period × 1.615m) × (resistance (kg) × 9.8)

Note: The distance for each revolution of the flywheel = 1.615m

Classification in terms of the results related to the peak power output can then be found using table 8.5.

2. Relative peak power output (RPP)

A more useful measure of peak power used to compare athletes or changes over time is to calculate peak power based on the subject's body mass. Peak power output relative to body mass is calculated as follows:

RPP = PP/body mass (kg)

Relative peak power ranges from as low as $6W.kg^{-1}$ in untrained females to $16W.kg^{-1}$ in some male athletes.

Classification in terms of the results related to the relative peak power output can be found using table 8.5.

Table 8.5	Percentile normative data for absolute and relative peak power and fatigue index for active young adults (Maud and Shultz 1989)					
	Absolute		Relative		Fatigue index	
	Male	Female	Male	Female	Male	Female
%Rank	W	W	W/kg	W/kg	(%)	(%)
90	822	560	10.89	9.02	51.7	47.3
80	777	527	10.39	8.83	46.7	43.6
70	757	505	10.20	8.53	43.5	40.3
60	721	480	9.80	8.14	39.9	38.2
50	689	449	9.22	7.65	38.4	35.2
40	671	432	8.92	6.96	35.0	33.7
30	656	399	8.53	6.86	31.1	28.7
20	618	376	8.24	6.57	29.6	26.5
10	570	353	7.06	5.98	23.2	25

Note: Peak power outputs of over 2,200 W have been reported in sprint cyclists such as Chris Hoy.

3. Anaerobic capacity (AC)

The sources of energy during a 30-second Wingate test are typically 50–55 per cent from anaerobic glycolysis, 23–29 per cent from the phosphagen system and 16–25 per cent from the aerobic system. Some of the criticism of the WAnT as a measure of anaerobic capacity is that it is not entirely anaerobic, and also not long enough to achieve full depletion of anaerobic energy sources. Despite this, some investigators have proposed the use of data from Wingate testing to estimate anaerobic capacity.

For total work accomplished in 30 seconds, anaerobic capacity is calculated as follows:

$$AC = \text{sum of each 5-second PP or}$$

$$AC = \text{force} \times \text{total distance in 30 seconds}$$

More recent studies show that the total average workload maintained over the 30-second period is not a good predictor of anaerobic capacity. They did, however, find that if WAnT is performed, then the subject's fatigue index was the best measure of anaerobic capacity. Remember, though, that fatigue index values depend on the length of the test performed.

4. Fatigue index (FI)

The *fatigue index* (discussed in chapter 7) can be described as the percentage decrease in power from peak to minimal power output, or in other words:

$$FI = [(\text{peak power} - \text{minimum power})/ \text{peak power}] \times 100\%$$

From the example of a 30-second WAnT in figure 8.11, peak power is 1200W and occurs after 2 seconds. Minimum power is obtained in the final 3 seconds and is 500W. Fatigue index for that subject can then be calculated as:

$$[(1200 - 500)/1200] \times 100\% = 58\%$$

In other words, this represents a decrease in peak power of 58 per cent over a 30-second period. Classification in terms of the results related to the fatigue index can be found using table 8.5.

Margaria-Kalamen step test

In previous years, stair climbing has been used as a method to estimate peak anaerobic power. The basic protocol of Margaria was first described in 1966 and updated by Kalamen two years later.

The test involves ascending a nine-step staircase of about 1.575 metres in height as rapidly as possible following a run-up of 6 metres. This step-test has been used for many years as a classic indicator of alactic anaerobic power (i.e. power of the phosphagen system).

The division between alactic and lactic anaerobic power output is questionable as, even in a test such as the Margaria-Kalamen step test, there would still be a significant contribution from anaerobic glycolysis (lactic system).

Required resources

Staircase with 12 steps, each 17.5cm high, the vertical distance between the 3rd and 9th step having been accurately measured; tape measure; weighing scales; stopwatch or timing mat/gates.

Testing method

1. Subject stands 6 metres from the start of the steps and sprints towards them on the command 'go'.
2. The subject then sprints up the flight of steps, three at a time, stepping on the 3rd, 6th and 9th steps.
3. The time to get from the 3rd to the 9th step should be accurately recorded, starting when the foot first contacts the third step and ending when it first contacts the 9th step.
4. Allow three trials with 2–3 minutes recovery between trials.

Analysis

To calculate the power developed as a result of this particular test, the following formula can be used:

$$\text{Power (W)} = \frac{\text{body mass (kg)} \times \text{vertical displacement (m)} \times 9.8}{\text{time (s)}}$$

So, for a 70kg individual running from step 3 to 9 in 0.6 seconds, their estimated power is: $(70 \times 1.05 \times 9.8)/0.6 = 1201\text{W}$

Classification

Even though there are no published normative data tables for this particular test, power outputs range from less than 700W in untrained females to as high as 1500W in trained males.

Table 8.6	Average peak and mean anaerobic values during a Bosco continuous jumping 60-second test	
	Peak anaerobic power (W)	Mean anaerobic power (W)
Male	1600	1200
Female	900	700

Bosco continuous jumping test

Anaerobic power has also been determined using a timing mat by the late Carmelo Bosco and colleagues (1983). In this test, subjects jump continuously for a certain time period of 30 or 60 seconds. Peak anaerobic power is determined as the highest maintained over a 5-second period.

Some of the advantages of the Bosco continuous jumping test are the relatively inexpensive equipment and the portability of the test. Similarly to Wingate testing, fatigue index can also be measured. The values obtained during continuous jumping are greater than those during Wingate testing, which may be due to the use of the greater power production of the stretch shortening cycle.

Care must be taken towards the end of the test, particularly in those less trained, as poor jump technique aligned with fatigue could increase injury risks.

Analysis

The peak and mean anaerobic power can be calculated using the formulas:

$$\text{Peak anaerobic power} =$$
$$(9.8 \times \text{total flight time (s)} \times 5)/[4 \times \text{number of jumps} \times (5 - \text{total flight time (s)})]$$

and:

$$\text{Mean anaerobic power (over a 60s period)} =$$
$$(9.8 \times \text{total flight time (s)} \times 60)/[4 \times \text{number of jumps} \times (60 - \text{total flight time (s)})]$$

Classification

Average values for both peak and mean anaerobic power during a 60-second test for active males and females can be seen in table 8.6.

Further reading

American College of Sports Medicine (2001) 'Position Statement: Plyometric training for children and adolescents'. Lippincott Williams & Wilkins, Indianapolis, Indiana

Ashley, C. (1994) 'Vertical jump performance and selected physiological characteristics of women'. *Journal of Strength and Conditioning Research*, 8: pp. 5-11

Baker, J. (2005) *Improving Jumping Performance: A brief overview.* Australian Institute of Sport Publications. Belconnen: Australia

Baker, J., Ramsbottom, R. & Hazeldine, R. (1993) 'Maximal shuttle running over 40m as a measure of anaerobic performance'. *British Journal of Sports Medicine*, 27: pp. 228-36

Bar-Or, O. (1987) 'The Wingate anaerobic test: An update on methodology, reliability and validity'. *Sports Medicine*, 4: pp. 381-94

Bauer, T. (1990) 'Comparison of training modalities for power development in the lower extremity'. *Journal of Applied Physiology*, 74: pp. 359-68

Beneke, R., Pollmann, C., Bleif, I., Leithauser, R. M. & Hutler, M. (2002) 'How anaerobic is the Wingate anaerobic test for humans?' *European Journal of Applied Physiology*, 87: pp. 388-92

Bosco, C., Luhtanen, P. & Komi, P. V., (1983) 'A simple method for measurement of mechanical power in jumping'. *European Journal of Applied Physiology*, 50: pp. 273-82

Canavan, P. K. & Vescovi, J. D. (2004) 'Evaluation of power prediction equations: Peak vertical jumping power in women'. *Medicine and Science in Sports and Exercise*, 36: pp. 1589-93

Chu, D. A. (1996) *Explosive power and strength: Complex training for maximum results,* Champaign, Illinois: Human Kinetics

Chu, D. A. (1998) *Jumping into Plyometrics*, 2nd edn, Champaign, Illinois: Human Kinetics

Coulson, M. & Archer, D. (2008) *Fitness Professionals: The Advanced Fitness Instructor's Handbook*, London, UK: A&C Black

Diallo, O., Dore, E., Duche, P. & Van Praagh, E. (2001) 'Effects of plyometric training followed by a reduced training programme on physical performance in prepubescent soccer players'. *Journal of Sports Medicine and Physical Fitness*, 41: pp. 342-8

Faria, E. W., Parker, D. L. & Faria, I. E. (2005) 'The science of cycling: Physiology and training – part 1'. *Sports Medicine*, 35: pp. 285-312

Harley, R. A. & Doust, J. H. (1997) *Strength and Fitness Training for Basketball: A sports science manual,* Leeds, UK: National Coaching Foundation

Harman, E. A., Rosenstein, M. T., Frykman, P. N., Rosenstein, R. M. & Kramer, W. J. (1991) 'Estimates of human power output from vertical jump'. *Journal of Applied Sport Science Research*, 5: pp. 116-20

Holcomb, W. R., Lander, J. E., Rutland, R. M. & Wilson, G. D. (1996) 'The effectiveness of a modified plyometric programme on power and the vertical jump'. *Journal of Strength and Conditioning Research*, 10: pp. 89-92

Inbar, O., Bar-Or, O. & Skinner, J. S. (1996) *The Wingate Anaerobic Test*, Champaign, Illinois: Human Kinetics

Kalamen, J. (1968) 'Measurement of maximum muscular power in man'. Doctoral thesis, Ohio State University

Linthorne, N. P. (2001) 'Analysis of standing vertical jumps using a force platform'. *American Journal of Physics*, 69: pp. 1198-1204

Luebbers, P. E., Potteiger, J. A., Hulver, M. W., Thyfault, J. P., Carper, M. J. & Lockwood, R. H. (2003) 'Effect of plyometric training and recovery on vertical jump performance and anaerobic power'. *Journal of Strength and Conditioning Research*, 17: pp. 704-9

Margaria, R., Aghmeo, P. & Rovelli, E. (1966) 'Measurement of muscular power (anaerobic) in man'. *Journal of Applied Physiology*, 21: pp. 1662-4

Masamoto, N., Larson, R., Gates, T. & Faigenbaum, A. (2003) 'Acute effects of plyometric exercise on maximum squat performance in male athletes'. *Journal of Strength and Conditioning Research*, 17: pp. 68-71

Maud, P. J. & Shultz, B. B. (1989) 'Norms for the Wingate anaerobic test with comparison to another similar test'. *Research Quarterly for Exercise and Sport*, 60: pp. 144-51

Micklewright, D., Alkhatib, A. & Beneke, R. (2006) 'Mechanically vs. electro-magnetically braked cycle ergometer: Performance and energy cost of the Wingate anaerobic test'. *European Journal of Applied Physiology*, 96: pp. 748-51

Minahan, C., Chia, M. & Inbar, O. (2007) 'Does power indicate capacity? 30-s Wingate anaerobic test vs. maximal accumulated O_2 deficit'. *International Journal of Sports Medicine*, 28: pp. 836-43

Sargent, D. A. (1921) 'The physical test of a man'. *American Physical Education Review*, 26: pp. 188-94

Sayers, S. P., Harackiewicz, D. V., Harman, E. A., Frykman, P. N. & Rosenstein, M. T. (1999) 'Cross-validation of three jump power equations'. *Medicine and Science in Sports and Exercise*, 31: pp. 572-7

Van Praagh, E. & França, N. M. (1998) 'Measuring maximal short-term power output during growth'. In Van Praagh, E. (ed.) *Pediatric Anaerobic Performance*, Champaign, Illinois: Human Kinetics, pp. 155-83

AEROBIC ENDURANCE TESTING

9

OBJECTIVES

After completing this chapter you should be able to:

1 Explain the term 'aerobic capacity' and state the units of measurement – relative and absolute.

2 Discuss the differences between direct and indirect tests and maximal and sub-maximal tests.

3 List and discuss a range of ergometers used for testing purposes.

4 Explain the use of gas analysers in direct testing methods.

5 Assess VO_2 max as a predictor of performance in sport.

6 List the factors affecting aerobic capacity.

7 Explain differences in VO_2 max values obtained during different modes of exercise – cycle ergometer versus treadmill.

8 Understand benefits and limitations of submaximal testing techniques and the variability in heart rate response to exercise between individuals.

9 Recognise validity of multistage fitness tests in assessing VO_2 max.

10 Outline the effect of environmental conditions on test results, particularly in field tests of aerobic endurance.

VO_2 max

At rest or when exercising, the volume of oxygen consumed is mainly dependent on the intensity of the activity. As the exercise intensity increases, the volume of oxygen consumed increases directly until it reaches a plateau as in figure 9.1. This plateau, or peak value, is termed VO_2 *max* and is also commonly known as *aerobic capacity, aerobic power* or *maximal oxygen uptake.*

Essentially this is a measurement of the maximum amount of oxygen used in litres per minute. This maximum amount is known as *absolute* VO_2 *max* and is commonly measured in sports such as rowing where body mass is supported when exercising. In many sports where body mass is not supported, for example running or cycling, VO_2 max is more commonly reported relative to body mass. This can be stated as millilitres of oxygen used in one minute per kilogram of bodyweight $(mlO_2.kg^{-1}.min^{-1})$. When measured relative to bodyweight, this is termed *relative* VO_2 *max* (see fig. 9.2 for typical values).

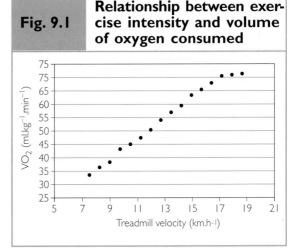

Fig. 9.1 Relationship between exercise intensity and volume of oxygen consumed

VO_2 (ml.kg^{-1}.min^{-1}) vs Treadmill velocity (km.h-1)

Fig. 9.2 | **Typical maximal oxygen uptake levels**

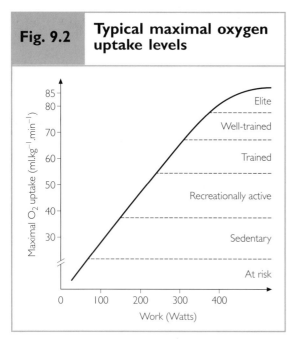

Fig. 9.3 | **Types of VO₂ testing**

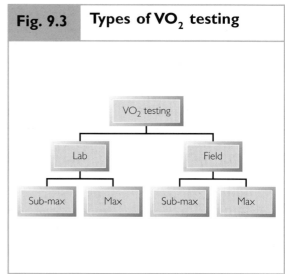

Testing can be done either at sub-maximal levels or at maximum capability, depending on the experience of the individual being tested, the experience of the tester and the goal of the test. Testing to maximum levels or capability is referred to as a VO_2 max test.

There are two general classifications of VO_2 testing, known as *direct* and *indirect* testing. Direct testing involves using a method of collecting air breathed out by the individual or subject (breath by breath) and then analysing that air content for volume and for oxygen and carbon dioxide concentration. This is known as *respiratory gas analysis.* Equipment needed for gas analysis can be used both in a laboratory setting and in a field setting, if portable. This type of equipment is not readily available to the general public as it is expensive and requires constant calibration, so a number of indirect VO_2 tests have been devised.

Some indirect tests are classed as maximal tests (subjects are taken to maximum capability);

however, there are many sub-maximal tests available that allow for the *estimation* of VO_2 max. Some of the indirect methods of testing for VO_2 include the Conconi test, Cooper test, Balke test, multi-stage fitness test (also known as the bleep test) and the Rockport walking test. These tests do not directly measure the amount of oxygen taken into and used by the muscle tissue. The score from the test is, however, converted to $mlO_2.kg^{-1}.min^{-1}$ so that this figure can be referenced against one of the score tables (normative value tables).

A complete gas analysis set-up would cost approximately £8,000–£10,000, which is beyond the budgets of most individuals. However, some university departments hire out laboratories or portable equipment to individuals. A typical charge for a VO_2 max test is in the region of £60–70 and closer to £100 if lactate threshold testing is included. However, university researchers are often looking for subjects to take part in experiments in exercise physiology and, depending on the nature of the project, direct VO_2 max testing may be part of the procedure. Directing an athlete to the local sport science department might be a first step in gaining useful information such as VO_2 max or economy of movement. It would be advisable, though, to be able to understand how this data was collected and be able to interpret it, so it is important to understand some of the basics about how direct VO_2 max testing is performed and the principles behind it.

The cardiovascular and respiratory systems are activated during exercise, providing oxygen to working muscles, and removing by-products of metabolism, such as carbon dioxide. Collection and analysis of respiratory gas samples during exercise is a fundamental part of an investigation in exercise physiology testing. Based on these data, several important measures can be made:

1. Determination of maximal oxygen uptake (VO_2 max)
2. Ventilatory threshold (see chapter 10)
3. Economy of movement (running, rowing, swimming etc.)
4. Fuel utilisation (fats/carbohydrates)
5. Resting metabolic rate (RMR)

The first four measures are an important component of aerobic fitness and the final measure, RMR, is useful in calculating an individual's energy requirements. These measurements can be used to examine an individual's potential for aerobic exercise, set training intensities and assess the effectiveness of training.

Ergometers

An ergometer is a machine that can measure the work performed during an exercise test. There are several types of ergometer, such as a treadmill, cycle or rower, but it is important that the ones used are safe and regularly calibrated. To minimise variation between ergometers, it might be useful to record which ergometer the subject was tested on and to continue to use that type if possible.

Cycle ergometers

Most exercise testing is performed on Monark cycle ergometers. These cost in the range of £1,000 to £2,000, depending on the model. If properly maintained and serviced regularly, they are capable of a long life. Servicing minimises the frictional load of the transmission and involves lubricating the chain, checking the ball bearings and adjusting the chain.

Monark cycle ergometers have a mechanical brake and the workload is based on the friction on the flywheel resulting from the total mass of the balance (see figure 9.4). A simple way to calculate the workload (W) when using the cycle is to multiply the total mass of the balance

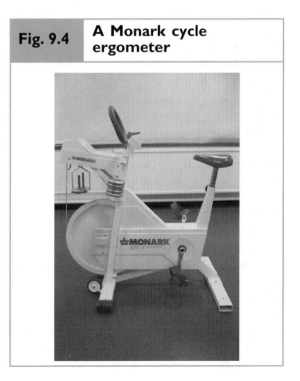

Fig. 9.4 **A Monark cycle ergometer**

(remember that the balance itself will weigh either 0.5 or 1.0kg) by the pedal cadence (revolution speed).

Therefore, cycling at 60rpm with a total mass of 2kg, including the balance, is equivalent to cycling at 120W. Close attention to cadence has to be made when testing on mechanically-braked ergometers since subjects will often decrease their cadence as they start to fatigue (resulting in incorrect workloads).

Electromechanically-braked cycle ergometers are more expensive than mechanically-braked, but have some advantages. The workload can be set independent of the pedal cadence and thus the subject can vary the cadence themselves. The Netherlands-based company Lode has manufactured a wide variety of electromechanically-braked cycle ergometers since 1952 and prices start around £6,000 for the Corival. Other ergometers such as the KingCycle ergometer use the subject's own personal cycle, which is attached to a test rig. The back wheel of the bike powers a roller, which is connected to a fan to create air resistance. KingCycle ergometers are usually cheaper than electromechanically-braked cycle ergometers. Another more recent development is the mobile ergometer; whereby a specialist device known as an SRM crank can be fitted to the drive chain of the subject's own cycle to give direct readings of torque and power output. Powertap hubs are another similar system, connected to the hub of the bike, and are less expensive than SRM cranks.

Treadmills

Some treadmills can be more comfortable for the subject to run on than others. For example, the Woodway treadmill is more comfortable and puts less stress on the joints than a treadmill with less cushioning. However, it is important that all treadmills are regularly calibrated.

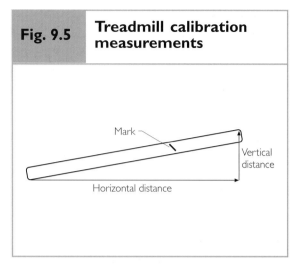

Fig. 9.5 Treadmill calibration measurements

Calibration of treadmills can be performed by marking a line on the belt, measuring the total belt length, and counting the revolutions per minute to calculate the speed. Percentage gradient can be assessed as the vertical height at the top of the belt divided by the horizontal distance (see figure 9.5) and multiplied by 100. The gradient should be within 0.1 per cent and speed within $0.1km.h^{-1}$ of the displayed values. Other issues such as belt slippage can also adversely affect treadmill reliability.

Rowing and kayak ergometers

Concept II ergometers are the most commonly used ergometers worldwide and are used to test rowers. Calibration is within 2 per cent of the measured power output and there are two models available – Concept IID and Concept IIE, both of which are considered very robust. The IID model is less expensive than the IIE and for home use would be a more suitable choice. There are several kayak ergometers available on the market such as KayakPro and Vasa Kayak Ergometer, which cost around £1,500.

Direct VO₂ max testing

VO_2 max testing can be either *continuous* (no rest between stages) or *discontinuous* (several minutes rest between stages). The choice may depend on the equipment and the number of staff available. If automated gas analysis equipment is available, it is not as demanding for a single investigator to perform continuous tests as it would to be using the Douglas bag method.

Douglas bags

Testing by the Douglas bag method was developed nearly 100 years ago, but is still considered by many to be the gold standard to which all other tests are compared. This type of testing is also known as open-circuit spirometry. With this method, expired gas (air breathed out) is collected in Douglas bags (see figure 9.6a) over a timed period (usually 60 seconds) and analysed for the following:

- Oxygen concentration (FEO_2); %
- Carbon dioxide concentration ($FECO_2$); %
- Gas volume (V_E); litres
- Ambient barometric pressure (P_a); mmHg
- Gas temperature (T_g); °C

Subjects are required to wear a mouthpiece and a nose clip during testing. The mouthpiece is attached to a two-way valve, such as manufactured by Hans Rudolphe (see figure 9.6b), ensuring no gases are lost.

Oxygen and carbon dioxide concentration is measured by passing a small volume of air through a gas analyser such as the Servomex 1440 for 30–60 seconds. The volume of air required for this analysis should be accounted for in calculations of bag volume. The bag is then evacuated through a dry-gas volume meter,

such as the Parkinson-Cowan, and volume recorded. Gas temperature is recorded by a thermistor attached to the tubing of the volume meter. Ambient pressure can be obtained from a mercury or aneroid barometer.

Placing the measured parameters into a spreadsheet or calculating them by hand gives volume of oxygen consumed (VO_2), volume of carbon dioxide produced (VCO_2), ventilation (V_E) and respiratory exchange ratio (RER) (see appendix to this chapter, p. 208).

Gas analysers should be calibrated before each test session with gases of known concentration. Room air is often used as the upper standard for oxygen, with an oxygen percentage of 20.93. Nitrogen is often used as a zero standard for both oxygen and carbon dioxide. Volume meters should be regularly calibrated through the use of a 3-litre syringe.

The total error of measurement in VO_2 max testing using Douglas bags is approximately

Fig. 9.6a	**Douglas bag set-up**

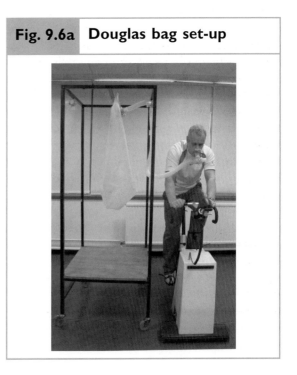

Fig. 9.6b Hans Rudolphe valve

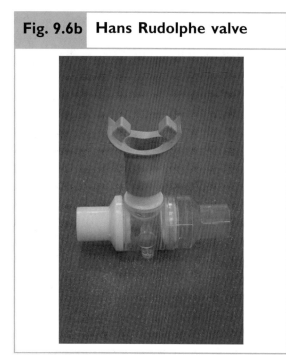

1.5 per cent and biological variation is approximately 2.0 per cent. The greatest potential for error comes from the measurement of oxygen concentration (a 1 per cent overestimation of expired oxygen concentration will result in a 5 per cent underestimate of VO_2 max).

Some of the limitations of the Douglas bag method are that leakages may occur or gases may become trapped during evacuation. Although rapid changes in V_E or VO_2 cannot be measured using Douglas bags unless bags are changed frequently, this is the most accurate method to determine VO_2 max. The main disadvantage is that the process is more time-consuming than automated gas analysis set-ups.

Automated gas analysis systems

Rather than testers having to collect and analyse the gas manually, manufacturers have developed automated systems, also known as metabolic carts. There are more than a dozen manufacturers of automated online gas analysers.

The principle behind automated analysers is the same as for the Douglas bag method. The volume of air inspired is measured by a low-resistance turbine or ultrasonic flow-meter. A sample of inspired gas is analysed for oxygen and carbon dioxide (see figure 9.7a).

One problem with many automated analysers is that volume is measured immediately but there is a delay with the measurement of O_2 and CO_2 concentrations. Calculations within the software attempt to match up the correct volume with the correct O_2 and CO_2 concentrations. Flow-meter accuracy is between 1 and 2 per cent (1 per cent for volumes greater than 100 litres and 2 per cent for volumes below 100 litres).

The error involved in measuring VO_2 max is greater for automated gas analysers than for the Douglas bag method and amounts to 5–10 per cent. Overestimates of true VO_2 max from

Fig. 9.7a Online gas analysis

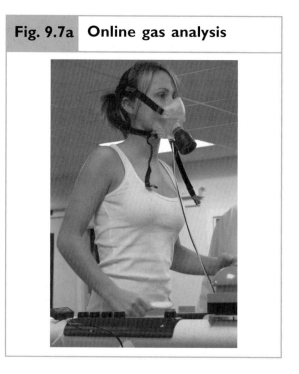

automated gas analysers are more common than underestimates. Repeated testing of a subject should be performed using the same analyser to minimise variability in VO_2 max values obtained.

A further development is the use of portable online gas analysers such as the Cortex Metamax 3B (see figure 9.7b) or Cosmed K4b2, which can be used for field testing. Rather than measuring VO_2 on a rowing ergometer, it can be measured while rowing on the water. Prices of these analysers are approximately £8,000–12,000.

Fig. 9.7b	Portable gas analyser

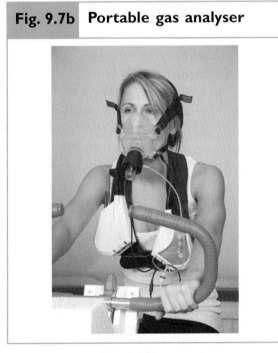

Protocols for VO_2 max

The mode of exercise can affect the VO_2 max values obtained, as differences in VO_2 max mainly reflect the quantity of muscle mass activated during the exercise. Treadmill testing tends to produce the greatest VO_2 max values, particularly in those more accustomed to running than cycling. Arm-cranking exercises typically produce VO_2 max values around 30 per cent below those obtained from cycling, and swimming produces VO_2 max values 20 per cent below those obtained in treadmill testing.

These differences between modes of exercise are lower in those who are trained in that particular mode of exercise. For example, trained cyclists achieve VO_2 max values that are similar to those they obtain on a treadmill, and trained swimmers achieve VO_2 max values that are only 10 per cent lower than they record on a treadmill. Also, VO_2 max values obtained on a cycle ergometer tend to be lower than treadmill testing as local muscle fatigue can occur in the quadriceps and hamstrings in those who are unaccustomed to cycling, causing them to cease exercising before a true VO_2 max is reached.

Test durations of between 8 and 12 minutes, with one-minute increments of approximately 25W, produce the greatest VO_2 max values. If lactate threshold testing is desired, 3 to 4-minute stages must be used and hence VO_2 max values are often marginally lower due to the longer test duration.

For experienced cyclists, subjects should be allowed to use higher cadences (90–100rpm) than for standard VO_2 max testing (60rpm). Starting workloads should be between 150 and 175W for males and 100W for females, with an increase of 25W per minute. The workload or treadmill velocity at which VO_2 max is reached is as important as the VO_2 max obtained and is often better correlated with performance than VO_2 max. In experienced cyclists this will be over 300W and 400W in males and females, respectively.

Bruce protocol

The Bruce protocol tends to be the most commonly used for testing patients with heart disease. The protocol (table 9.1) has seven 3-minute stages, resulting in 21 minutes of exercise. Starting treadmill speed is 1.7mph (2.7km.h^{-1}) at 10 per cent gradient. Clinical subjects rarely complete the test; however, 9–12 minutes of exercise is usually enough for subjects to reach 85 per cent of maximum predicted heart rate and is sufficient to assess cardiac functioning. The most common reason for cessation of an exercise test in this population is fatigue and breathlessness (dyspnea) as a result of being unaccustomed to the exercise.

Table 9.1	Bruce protocol		
Time (min)	Treadmill speed (mph)	Treadmill speed (km.h^{-1})	Treadmill gradient (%)
0–3	1.7	2.7	10
3–6	2.5	4.0	12
6–9	3.4	5.5	14
9–12	4.2	6.8	16
12–15	5.0	8.0	18
15–18	5.5	8.9	20
18–21	6.0	9.7	22

Balke protocol

The Balke test is a widely used graded exercise test performed on a treadmill. Starting speed is initially set at 3.3mph (5.3km.h^{-1}) with a gradient of 0 per cent (table 9.2). The speed is then kept constant and the gradient increases to 2 per cent at the end of the first minute. The gradient then increases by 1 per cent per minute until 25 per cent is reached. Thereafter the gradient is kept constant and speed is increased by 0.2mph

(0.32km.h^{-1}) every minute until exhaustion. VO$_2$ max values obtained from the Bruce protocol tend to be higher than those obtained from the Balke protocol. However, in subjects with low fitness level, true VO$_2$ max values can be obtained, but in fitter individuals, the duration of the test is often too long.

Table 9.2	Balke protocol		
Time (min)	Treadmill speed (mph)	Treadmill speed (km.h^{-1})	Treadmill gradient (%)
0–1	3.3	5.3	0
1–2	3.3	5.3	2
3–4	3.3	5.3	3
4–5	3.3	5.3	4
25–26	3.3	5.3	25
26–27	3.5	5.6	25
28–29	3.7	5.9	25
Exhaustion	Exhaustion	Exhaustion	25

Criteria for a subject achieving VO$_2$ max

There are several situations in which the investigator can assume that the subject being tested has reached the point of VO$_2$ max. The main criteria are considered to be the following:

1. Plateau in VO$_2$, despite increases in exercise intensity.
2. Blood lactate concentration > 8.0mmol.l^{-1} in first 5 minutes of recovery.
3. RER > 1.10.
4. HR $> 90\%$ age-predicted maximum.

A plateau in VO_2 is considered to be the main criterion for a subject reaching VO_2 max, but this generally occurs in only about 50 per cent of subjects in graded exercise tests. Many investigators accept a subject has reached VO_2 max if two of the other three criteria are reached. If this is not the case then the outcome of the test should be termed VO_2 peak rather than VO_2 max. If VO_2 max is not reached, a second testing session may be required within two to three days, starting exercise just below the peak workloads reached in the first test.

Classification

There are many classification tables available for specific age, gender and other such parameters. Table 9.3 shows classifications for general populations related to gender and age. These normative-value classifications can be used to classify subjects for all tests (not just the ones within this book) of VO_2 max.

Maximal indirect tests of VO_2 max

Multi-stage fitness test

The multi-stage fitness test (commonly referred to as the bleep test) is thought to be a reliable and efficient means of testing maximal oxygen uptake outside the laboratory. Brewer and

Table 9.3	Male and female normative values for VO_2					
Female (values in $mlO_2.kg^{-1}.min^{-1}$)						
Age	Very poor	Poor	Fair	Good	Excellent	Superior
13–19	<25.0	25.0–30.9	31.0–34.9	35.0–38.9	39.0–41.9	>41.9
20–29	<23.6	23.6–28.9	29.0–32.9	33.0–36.9	37.0–41.0	>41.0
30–39	<22.8	22.8–26.9	27.0–31.4	31.5–35.6	35.7–40.0	>40.0
40–49	<21.0	21.0–24.4	24.5–28.9	29.0–32.8	32.9–36.9	>36.9
50–59	<20.2	20.2–22.7	22.8–26.9	27.0–31.4	31.5–35.7	>35.7
>59	<17.5	17.5–20.1	20.2–24.4	24.5–30.2	30.3–31.4	>31.4
Male (values in $mlO_2.kg^{-1}.min^{-1}$)						
Age	Very poor	Poor	Fair	Good	Excellent	Superior
13–19	<35.0	35.0–38.3	38.4–45.1	45.2–50.9	51.0–55.9	>55.9
20–29	<33.0	33.0–36.4	36.5–42.4	42.5–46.4	46.5–52.4	>52.4
30–39	<31.5	31.5–35.4	35.5–40.9	41.0–44.9	45.0–49.4	>49.4
40–49	<30.2	30.2–33.5	33.6–38.9	39.0–43.7	43.8–48.0	>48.0
50–59	<26.1	26.1–30.9	31.0–35.7	35.8–40.9	41.0–45.3	>45.3
>59	<20.5	20.5–26.0	26.1–32.2	32.3–36.4	36.5–44.2	>44.2

colleagues also found a good correlation between performance in the multi-stage fitness test and the time to complete a 5km run, and Paliczka and colleagues found a similar relationship for a 10km run.

The acceleration and deceleration involved in the multi-stage fitness test is more specific to the patterns of movement in team sports than constant speed running in graded exercise tests on a treadmill. Due to the changes in direction involved, this test would not be recommended for use on middle- or long-distance runners, whose pacing is kept relatively constant during competition.

Many subjects can be tested at once; one tester can test up to six subjects at a time.

Required resources

A flat, non-slippery surface at least 20 metres in length; 30-metre tape measure; marking cones; pre-recorded audio tape or CD; tape recorder or CD player.

Testing method

The test is made up of 23 exercise levels where each lasts approximately one minute. Each level comprises a series of 20-metre shuttle runs where the starting speed is 8.5km.hr^{-1} and increases by 0.5km.hr^{-1} at each level. On the tape, a single bleep indicates the end of a shuttle and three bleeps indicates the start of the next level. The protocol for conducting the test is as follows:

1. Measure out a 20-metre section on a flat surface with a marker cone or line at each end.
2. The subjects carry out a warm-up programme of jogging and stretching exercises.
3. The test is then started after all subjects have been given clear instructions.
4. The subjects must place one foot on or beyond the 20-metre marker at the end of each shuttle.

5. If a subject arrives at the end of a shuttle before the bleep, they must wait for the bleep and then resume running.
6. Subjects are to keep running for as long as possible until they can no longer keep up with the speed set by the tape bleeps. At this point they withdraw.
7. Issue a warning if a subject fails to reach the end of the shuttle before the bleep. They should be allowed two or three further shuttles to attempt to regain the required pace before being withdrawn. Record the level attained.

Analysis

Use table 9.4 to estimate the VO$_2$ max score from the highest level achieved by the subject, then use table 9.3 to find the classification.

In the authors' experience of testing professional footballers for VO$_2$ max (among other parameters), outfield players typically reach between level 12 and level 15 on the multi-stage fitness test.

Professional rugby players typically reach between levels 12 and 13, although there are position differences within this sport as back players tend to reach greater values than forward players, probably due to their greater aerobic fitness and lower body mass.

It has also been found that VO$_2$ max values range between 50 and 60ml.kg^{-1}.min^{-1} for rugby union players. As a general rule, rugby union and basketball players' VO$_2$ max values tend to be lower than for other sports individuals such as field hockey or soccer players.

Like all maximal testing, though, accurate values are dependent on subjects giving a maximal effort throughout the test.

The multi-stage fitness test has been used for over 20 years as a means of testing subjects within team sports. One of the main limitations of the test is that it is not fully representative of the activity patterns displayed in most team sports. In soccer,

Table 9.4	Multi-stage fitness test levels and VO_2max scores				
Level	Shuttle	VO_2 max	Level	Shuttle	VO_2 max
4	2	26.8	5	2	30.2
4	4	27.6	5	4	31.0
4	6	28.3	5	6	31.8
4	9	29.5	5	9	32.9
Level	Shuttle	VO_2 max	Level	Shuttle	VO_2 max
6	2	33.6	7	2	37.1
6	4	34.3	7	4	37.8
6	6	35.0	7	6	38.5
6	8	35.7	7	8	39.2
6	10	36.4	7	10	39.9
Level	Shuttle	VO_2 max	Level	Shuttle	VO_2 max
8	2	40.5	9	2	43.9
8	4	41.1	9	4	44.5
8	6	41.8	9	6	45.2
8	8	42.4	9	8	45.8
8	11	43.3	9	11	46.8
Level	Shuttle	VO_2 max	Level	Shuttle	VO_2 max
10	2	47.4	11	2	50.8
10	4	48.0	11	4	51.4
10	6	48.7	11	6	51.9
10	8	49.3	11	8	52.5
10	11	50.2	11	10	53.1
Level	Shuttle	VO_2 max	Level	Shuttle	VO_2 max
12	2	54.3	13	2	57.6
12	4	54.8	13	4	58.2
12	6	55.4	13	6	58.7

Table 9.4	Multi-stage fitness test levels and VO$_2$max scores (cont.)				
Level	Shuttle	VO$_2$ max	Level	Shuttle	VO$_2$ max
12	8	56.0	13	8	59.3
12	10	56.5	13	10	59.8
12	12	57.1	13	13	60.6
Level	Shuttle	VO$_2$ max	Level	Shuttle	VO$_2$ max
14	2	61.1	15	2	64.6
14	4	61.7	15	4	65.1
14	6	62.2	15	6	65.6
14	8	62.7	15	8	66.2
14	10	63.2	15	10	66.7
14	13	64.0	15	13	67.5
Level	Shuttle	VO$_2$ max	Level	Shuttle	VO$_2$ max
16	2	68.0	17	2	71.4
16	4	68.5	17	4	71.9
16	6	69.0	17	6	72.4
16	8	69.5	17	8	72.9
16	10	69.9	17	10	73.4
16	12	70.5	17	12	73.9
16	14	70.9	17	14	74.4
Level	Shuttle	VO$_2$ max	Level	Shuttle	VO$_2$ max
18	2	74.8	19	2	78.3
18	4	75.3	19	4	78.8
18	6	75.8	19	6	79.2
18	8	76.2	19	8	79.7
18	10	76.7	19	10	80.2
18	12	77.2	19	12	80.6
18	15	77.9	19	15	81.3

Table 9.4	Multi-stage fitness test levels and VO$_2$max scores (cont.)				
Level	Shuttle	VO$_2$ max	Level	Shuttle	VO$_2$ max
20	2	81.8	21	2	85.2
20	4	82.2	21	4	85.6
20	6	82.6	21	6	86.1
20	8	83.0	21	8	86.5
20	10	83.5	21	10	86.9
20	12	83.9	21	12	87.4
20	14	84.3	21	14	87.8
20	16	84.8	21	16	88.2

Table 9.5	Typical stages and predicted VO$_2$ max values reached by athletes performing the multi-stage fitness test		
Sport	Position	Level of shuttle	Predicted VO$_2$ max (ml.kg^{-1}.min^{-1})
Soccer	Outfield (male)	13–10 to15–10	60–67
Field hockey	Outfield (male)	14–5	62
Rugby union	Forward (male)	12–4	55
Rugby union	Back (male)	13–10	60
Rugby league	Forward (male)	13–10	60
Rugby league	Back (male)	14–6	62
Basketball	(Male)	11–5	52
Basketball	(Female)	9–6	45
Cricket	Test squad (male)	12–4	55
Cricket	Test squad (female)	10–6	49

for instance, players change directions or speeds every few seconds and have on average 72 seconds between sprints (Premier League players cover an average of 10.7km over a 90 minute match). An alternative to predicting VO$_2$ max using the bleep test is to measure performance in activities that replicate the physiological demands of competitive football, such as the yo-yo test devised by Bangsbo.

Intermittent yo-yo endurance test

This particular test was developed by Jens Bangsbo and follows a similar principle to that of the multi-stage fitness test. The set-up for this test can be seen in figure 9.8.

The difference between this test and the multi-stage fitness test is that at the end of each 2×20-metre run there is a brief 5-second period of active recovery (2×5-metre walk) before the next level.

The test can be performed at two settings, differing by the starting speed ($10km.h^{-1}$ on level one and $13km.h^{-1}$ on level two). Level one is suitable for less well-trained soccer players and lasts between 6 and 20 minutes. Level two is suitable for well-trained male soccer players and lasts between 2 and 10 minutes. The average distance covered during this test by under-19 and senior English Premiership footballers is approximately 2km.

As well as the intermittent test, Bangsbo also devised the recovery test. The principles of the yo-yo intermittent recovery test are the same as the intermittent yo-yo endurance test, except recovery times are 10 seconds. The distance covered during this test has been shown to be related to the subject's VO_2 max and distance covered when running at high intensity ($>15km.h^{-1}$) during a match.

Loughborough intermittent shuttle test (LIST)

Considered to be a similar test to the yo-yo test, although demanding more preparation time, is the LIST. The test is also performed over a 20-metre distance with running at varying speeds including maximal sprinting.

Part A of the test is represented by five 15-minute exercise periods separated by 3 minutes of recovery, and Part B of the test is represented by intermittent running to the point of exhaustion. The primary outcome measures of performance are the total distance covered and the run duration from Part B.

Some of the limitations of the LIST are that an initial multi-stage fitness test must be performed in order to set the intensities to be used, and that the test duration is relatively long (on average 85 minutes).

No VO_2 max values are obtained as a result of this test, but it is a useful soccer-specific test commonly used to measure aerobic endurance.

Astrand treadmill test

This is a maximal test designed for use with a treadmill. Informed consent must be given before a subject is allowed to perform the test.

Required resources

Treadmill with gradient, stopwatch.

Testing method

1. The treadmill is set up at the start with a speed of $8.05km.hr^{-1}$ (5mph) and no gradient.
2. The subject then commences the test.
3. After three minutes the gradient is set to 2.5 per cent.
4. After every two minutes the gradient is increased by 2.5 per cent as can be seen in table 9.6.

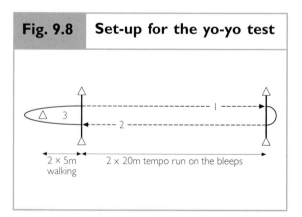

| Fig. 9.8 | Set-up for the yo-yo test |

2 × 5m walking
2 × 20m tempo run on the bleeps

Table 9.6	Astrand protocol
Time (min)	Treadmill gradient (%)
0–3	0
3–5	2.5
5–7	5
7–9	7.5
9–11	10
11–13	12.5
13–15	15
15–17	17.5
17–19	20
19–21	22.5
21–23	25
23–25	27.5
25–27	30
27–29	32.5
29–30	35

5. The tester should start the stopwatch at the beginning of the test and stop it when the subject is unable to continue.

Analysis

From the running time, the subject's VO_2 max can be calculated as follows:

$$VO_2 \text{ max} = (\text{time} \times 1.444) + 14.99$$

Time is the total time of the entire test expressed in minutes and fractions of a minute.

Sub-maximal testing

There are many field and laboratory tests, which have been developed over the years, that only require subjects to perform at sub-maximal heart rate levels; many individuals would not be suited to performing at maximal heart rate levels. As a result, these tests always involve predictions based on certain parameters such as heart rate or VO_2 max. If true maximum heart rate of the subject is known, some of the tests are considered to be reasonably accurate.

Predictions based on sub-maximal heart rate and VO_2

In laboratory-based situations, when time does not allow for a full VO_2 max test, or the subject does not elect to work at maximal levels, VO_2 max can be predicted based on the heart rate (HR) and VO_2 response to a period of increasing exercise intensity.

There is a direct linear relationship between HR and oxygen consumption (VO_2) during exercise, as can be seen in figure 9.9. By measuring heart rate and oxygen consumption at three increasing sub-maximal workloads (the intensity should be increased linearly), it is possible to extrapolate that line to the predicted HR max in order to predict VO_2 max of the subject being tested. Results for the subject in figure 9.9a show a predicted VO_2 max of 5.0l.min^{-1}. The data from the test subject could then be used to set exercise intensities for their training.

Take the example in figure 9.9b where an intensity equivalent to that of 60 per cent VO_2 max (3.0 litres) is set for steady state rowing. If actual HR max of the subject is known, it improves the accuracy of this test, as predicted HR max can often be 10bpm more or less than true HR max.

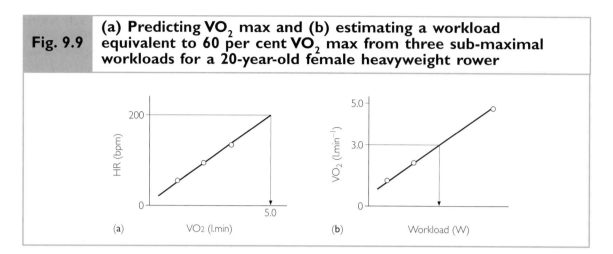

Fig. 9.9 **(a) Predicting VO$_2$ max and (b) estimating a workload equivalent to 60 per cent VO$_2$ max from three sub-maximal workloads for a 20-year-old female heavyweight rower**

(a) — HR (bpm) vs VO2 (l.min)

(b) — VO$_2$ (l.min^{-1}) vs Workload (W)

For testing of this kind the equipment must be regularly checked and calibrated for accuracy. It is also recommended that the equipment used for testing should be related to the sport or event of the subject being tested so that training intensities can be set for the training equipment that is normally used. Other than that, the resources required are a means of measuring heart rate and a method of recording and analysing the test results.

Harvard step test

The basis of this test is the assumption that the heart rate response to exercise is directly related to oxygen consumption. However, the heart rate response to a fixed-intensity bout of exercise would be lower in a more aerobically fit individual (i.e. they would be further from their maximum heart rate). This predicted VO$_2$ max is normally considered to be within 16 per cent of the true value for the Harvard step test.

This particular test is simple to administer but one of the limitations of this test for athletic populations is that the nature of the exercise is not very representative of typical movements in most sports, so it might be more suitable for a non-athletic population.

Required resources

Bench of appropriate height, metronome, heart rate monitor.

Fig. 9.10 **Extended leg during Harvard step test**

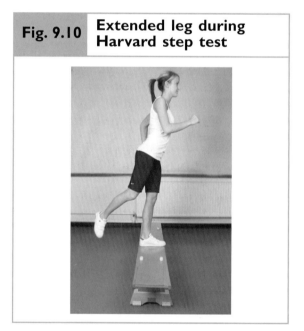

Testing method

The protocol for conducting the Harvard step test is as follows:

1. The subject steps on to a bench with one leg, then the other and then steps down in the same manner. They should fully extend the legs at the top of the step (see figure 9.10).
2. The step rate is set at 22 full steps (up, up, down, down) per minute for females and 24 steps per minute for males.
3. Subjects must maintain this stepping rate for three minutes with the step height always set at 41.3cm (16.25 inches).
4. After three minutes stepping, the subject remains standing.
5. The heart rate is then taken for a period of 15 seconds.
6. This number is multiplied by four to convert the heart rate to beats per minute.

Analysis

Use the formulae below to estimate the VO_2 max, and then refer to table 9.3 for classification.

Men:

VO_2 max (ml.kg^{-1}.min^{-1})
= 111.33 – (0.42 × bpm)

Women:

VO_2 max (ml.kg^{-1}.min^{-1})
= 65.81 – (0.1847 × bpm)

Astrand-Rhyming cycle test

The Astrand-Rhyming cycle test was initially developed around 1954 specifically as a sub-maximal predictor of VO_2 max. The test was designed to be performed on a cycle ergometer. The basis of the test is similar to that of the Harvard step test in that the heart rate response to a fixed bout of exercise is measured and the results subsequently analysed.

The accuracy of this particular test is considered to be about 10 per cent, due to variations in the relationship between heart rate and VO_2. It is an easily administered test, which can be used with sedentary populations.

One of the main disadvantages of the Astrand-Rhyming cycle test is that it requires a cycle ergometer (but this machine can also be used in many other tests).

Required resources

Cycle ergometer, stopwatch, heart rate monitor.

Testing method

The protocol for the Astrand-Rhyming test can vary depending on the subject:

1. The cycle ergometer should first be set up for each subject at their correct seat height. The subject wears a heart rate monitor.
2. Select the starting workload depending on the subject's body mass, fitness level and gender. This is usually 100 to 150W for young males and between 100 and 125W for young females (the selected workload should aim to increase the heart rate to a level between 130 and 160 bpm).
3. Once the workload is selected the subject should then pedal at 60rpm for six minutes.
4. Monitor heart rate every minute and adjust the workload up or down 25W if a heart rate of between 130 and 160bpm is not reached after two minutes of exercise.
5. Record the heart rate of the subject and workload at the end of exercise.

Analysis

Use an Astrand-Rhyming nomogram to predict VO_2 max from the test results data. This is a fixed data sheet on which VO_2 max can be read directly by the continuation of drawn lines from other data on the sheet.

Field testing

Field tests can be a more practical way of estimating aerobic capacity when testing large populations of subjects or when time or equipment is limited. Runs of various distances or durations can be used to evaluate aerobic fitness.

Cooper 12-minute run

In 1963, Balke developed a field performance test using a 15-minute run to assess aerobic fitness of military personnel. In 1968 Cooper shortened the test to a 12-minute run. He reported a correlation of r = 0.90 (very good correlation) between the distance covered in 12 minutes and VO$_2$ max in 115 males (aged 17–52 years). When other populations have been used this correlation has been found to be around 0.70 (which is considered a good correlation).

The test involves an individual running at maximal pace for 12 minutes and measuring the total distance covered. This test is widely used due to the simplicity of administration and the few resources that are required.

Required resources

400-metre track marked every 100 metres, stopwatch.

Testing method

1. Explain the concept of pacing to the subject, i.e. that they will have to try to maintain their maximum possible pace for 12 minutes.
2. Instruct the subject to cover the longest possible distance in 12 minutes. Walking is permitted, but it is preferable to run.
3. The subject lines up on the starting line and starts running on the command of the tester, who starts the stopwatch at exactly the same time.
4. The tester should call out the time at regular intervals.
5. After 11 minutes the tester should count down the last minute for the subject.
6. After 12 minutes the tester should measure the total distance covered by the subject.

Analysis

As with many other tests, analysis of the results (distance covered in this case) of the Cooper run can be done by comparing them with the results of previous tests, or a classification can be found by using normative data (tables 9.7 or 9.8).

Having completed the test, an approximate estimation of the VO$_2$ max (in ml.kg^{-1}.min^{-1}) of

Table 9.7	Cooper run normative data for young subjects (values in metres)				
Age	Excellent	Above average	Average	Below average	Poor
Male 13–14	>2700	2400–2700	2200–2399	2100–2199	<2100
Female 13–14	>2000	1900–2000	1600–1899	1500–1599	<1500
Male 15–16	>2800	2500–2800	2300–2499	2200–2299	<2200
Female 15–16	>2100	2000–2100	1700–1999	1600–1699	<1600
Male 17–19	>3000	2700–3000	2500–2699	2300–2499	<2300
Female 17–19	>2300	2100–2300	1800–2099	1700–1799	<1700

Table 9.8	Cooper run normative data for older subjects (values in metres)				
Age	Excellent	Above average	Average	Below average	Poor
Male 20–29	>2800	2400–2800	2200–2399	1600–2199	<1600
Female 20–29	>2700	2200–2700	1800–2199	1500–1799	<1500
Male 30–39	>2700	2300–2700	1900–2299	1500–1899	<1500
Female 30–39	>2500	2000–2500	1700–1999	1400–1699	<1400
Male 40–49	>2500	2100–2500	1700–2099	1400–1699	<1400
Female 40–49	>2300	1900–2300	1500–1899	1200–1499	<1200
Male >50	>2400	2000–2400	1600–1999	1300–1599	<1300
Female >50	>2200	1700–2200	1400–1699	1100–1399	<1100

the individual can also be calculated by using Cooper's equation:

$$VO_2 \ max = (d_{12} - 505) \ / \ 45$$

Note: In Cooper's equation, d_{12} represents the distance (measured in metres) covered in 12 minutes.

> *Example*: For a well-trained subject who covers a distance of 3,200m in 12 minutes, predicted VO_2 max would be $[(3,200 - 505)/45] = 59.9$ml.kg^{-1}.min^{-1}.

For middle or long distance runners, the Cooper test is a valid measure of aerobic endurance. It can be used to test a large number of subjects at once and can encourage the competitive nature of athletes.

One of the limitations of the Cooper test is that pacing can become an issue and a common occurrence is that subjects start off too quickly and fatigue early in the test, resulting in lower VO_2 max predictions. For team sports players, one of the limitations of the Cooper test is that there are not the same changes in direction and pace that occur in normal game play. For these reasons a test involving changes in pace and direction such as the multi-stage fitness test or Bangsbo yo-yo endurance test would be superior.

Rockport fitness walking test

This test has been validated for use in college-age males and females and is based on the time taken to complete a 1-mile (1609m) walk, finishing heart rate, weight, age and gender.

Required resources

400-metre track, stopwatch.

Testing method

1. Record the weight of the subject.
2. The subject lines up on the starting line.
3. The subject starts walking on the command of the tester who starts the stopwatch at the same time.
4. The subject walks one mile as fast as possible.
5. Immediately on finishing the walk, record the heart rate (bpm) and the time to complete the one-mile walk.

Analysis

VO_2 max can be found by using the following equation:

$$VO_2 \text{ max} =$$

$$132.853 - (0.0769 \times BW) - (0.3877 \times age) +$$
$$(6.3150 \times gender) - (3.2649 \times time) - (0.1565 \times HR)$$

where:
gender = 0 (female) or 1 (male)
time = walk time in minutes to the
            nearest hundredth of a minute
HR = heart rate (bpm) at the end of the test
BW = body weight in kg
age = age in years

For example, a female subject aged 25 with a body mass of 65kg, finishing heart rate of 190bpm and a one-mile time of 12min 45sec (12.75min) results in:
VO_2 max = $132.853 - (0.0769 \times 65) - (0.3877 \times 25) + (6.3150 \times 0) - (3.2649 \times 12.75) - (0.1565 \times 190) = 46.8$ml.kg^{-1}.min^{-1}.

Another similar test is the UKK 2km-walk test, developed in Finland. The equations to calculate VO_2 max with this test are:

$$VO_2 \text{ max (males)} =$$
$$184.0 - (4.65 \times time) - (1.05 \times BMI) - (0.26 \times age) - (0.22 \times HR)$$

$$VO_2 \text{ max (females)} =$$
$$116.2 - (2.98 \times time) - (0.39 \times BMI) - (0.14 \times age) - (0.11 \times HR)$$

Both of these walking tests would be recommended for use in healthy non-athletic populations. For more active, trained individuals, the Cooper test might be more appropriate.

Appendix

Oxygen consumption calculation

The calculation of the volume of oxygen consumed (VO_2), volume of oxygen produced (VCO_2) and respiratory exchange ratio (RER) are outlined below.

There are many spreadsheets available to automate these calculations, but it is still useful to be able to calculate them by hand.

The oxygen consumption is calculated as the difference between the amount of oxygen inspired and the amount of oxygen expired:

VO_2 equation:
VO_2 = volume of oxygen inspired
        − volume of oxygen expired

$$VO_2 = V_IO_2 - V_EO_2 \quad \text{so} \quad VO_2 = (V_I \times F_IO_2) - (V_E \times F_EO_2)$$

where: V_I = inspired air volume
              F_IO_2 = fractional oxygen content
                       of inspired air
              V_E = expired air volume
              F_EO_2 = fractional oxygen content
                       of expired air

Since gas volumes in the laboratory are dependent on ambient temperature and pressure, and exhaled air is usually saturated (ATPS), in order to standardise conditions, Charles' Law and Boyle's Law are invoked and corrected for vapour pressure. If you correct, in the first place, for V_E, all other subsequent gas calculations will be at a standardised temperature pressure, dry (STPD). Tables of water vapour pressure in air at different temperatures are provided in table 9.9.

$$V_{STPD} = V_{ATPS} \left[273/(273 + T_G)\right]\left[(P_A - P_{H2O})/P_S\right]$$

where:

T_G	= expired gas temperature in Celsius
P_A	= ambient barometric pressure (mmHg)
P_{H2O}	= partial pressure of water vapour at ambient temperature
P_S	= standard barometric pressure (760mmHg)
$(273 + T_G)$	= absolute temperature in Kelvin
STPD factor	= $\left[273/(273 + T_G)\right]\left[(P_A - P_{H2O})/P_S\right]$
i.e. STPD factor	= $\left[273/(273 + T_G)\right]\left[(P_A - P_{H2O})/760\right]$

F_IO_2 is known (the O_2 content of room air is constant at 20.93%, or 0.2093 as a ratio), and V_E and F_EO_2 are measured on the sample collected. Where the respiratory exchange ratio is exactly one, the inspired and expired volumes are equal but, since this rarely occurs, a correction must be applied. Since N_2 is not normally absorbed, the amount of N_2 inhaled must be equal to the amount of N_2 exhaled. Thus, the inspired volume is calculated from the change in nitrogen concentration as follows:

$$V_I \times F_IN_2 = V_E \times F_EN_2$$

where: F_IN_2 = %N_2 in inspired air (assumed to be 0.7904)
F_EN_2 = %N_2 in expired air
F_EN_2 = 1 i.e.- $(F_EO_2 + F_ECO_2)$

Rearranging the equation to calculate V_I:

$$V_I = (V_E \times F_EN_2)/0.7904$$

The VO_2 equation can now be used to calcu-late VO_2 since all the values on the right-hand side are known.

Carbon dioxide production calculation

Using similar calculations, the volume of VCO_2 production can be calculated.

VCO_2 = Volume of carbon dioxide expired
– volume of carbon dioxide inspired, so ...

$$VCO_2 = V_ECO_2 - V_ICO_2$$

For room air, which contains 0.03 per cent CO_2, the following equation is appropriate:

$$VCO_2 = (V_E) \times (\text{fraction of } CO_2 \text{ in expired air}) - V_I(0.0003)$$

Respiratory exchange ratio calculation

The respiratory exchange ratio (RER) can be calculated as follows:

$$RER = VCO_2/VO_2$$

Table 9.9	Vapour pressure (P_{H2O}) of wet gas at laboratory temperatures		
T (°C)	P_{H2O} (mmHg)	T (°C)	P_{H2O} (mmHg)
18	15.5	24	22.4
19	16.5	25	23.8
20	17.5	26	25.2
21	18.7	27	26.7
22	19.8	28	28.4
23	21.1	29	30.0

Sample data collection sheet for VO_2 max testing

Data sheet: treadmill

Barometric pressure:_____ Date:_____ Name:_____

Sport:_____ Position/event/distance:_____

Age:_____ Height:_____ Body mass:_____

Time (min)	Tread grade (%)	Tread velocity (km/h)	Bag time (s)	RPE	HR	FEO$_2$ (%)	FECO$_2$ (%)	Meter vol (l)	Samp vol (l)	Ventilation (l)
Rest	0	0								

Results

Time (min)	STPD factor	V_E (l.min^{-1}) ATPS	V_E (l.min^{-1}) STPD	VO$_2$ (l.min^{-1})	VCO$_2$ (l.min^{-1})	RER	VO$_2$ (ml^{-1}.kg^{-1} min^{-1})	Blood lactate (mmol.l^{-1})
Rest								

Further reading

Amann, M., Subudhi, A. & Foster, C. (2004) 'Influence of testing protocol on ventilatory thresholds and cycling performance'. *Medicine and Science in Sports and Exercise*, 36: pp. 613-22

Astrand, P-O. & Rhyming, I. (1954) 'A nomogram for calculation of aerobic capacity (physical fitness) from pulse rate during submaximal work'. *Journal of Applied Physiology*, 7: pp. 218-21

Bangsbo, J. (1995) *Fitness Training in Football: A scientific approach*, Bagsværd, Denmark: HO Storm

Bangsbo, J. (1996) *Yo–Yo Test*, Bagsværd Denmark: HO Storm

Balke, B. & Ware, R.W. (1959) 'An experimental study of physical fitness of Air Force personnel'. *U.S. Armed Forces Medical Journal*, 10: pp. 675-88

Bradley, P. S., Sheldon, W., Wooster, B., Olsen, P., Boanas, P. & Krustrup, P. (2009) 'High-intensity running in English FA Premier League soccer matches'. *Journal of Sports Sciences*, 27: pp. 159-68

Brouha, L., Graybiel, A. & Heath, C. W. (1943) 'The step test: A simple method of measuring physical fitness for hard muscular work in adult men'. *Reviews of Canadian Biology*, 2: pp. 86-92

Bruce, R. A., Kusumi, F. & Hosmer, D. (1973) 'Maximal oxygen intake and monograph assessment of functional aerobic impairment in cardiovascular disease'. *American Heart Journal*, 85: pp. 545-62

Cooper, K. H. (1968) 'A means of assessing maximal oxygen intake'. *Journal of the American Medical Association*, 203: pp. 135-8

Drust, B., Reilly, T. & Cable, N. T. (2000) 'Physiological responses to laboratory-based soccer-specific intermittent and continuous exercise'. *Journal of Sports Sciences*, 18: pp. 885-92

Duthie, G. M., Pyne, D. & Hooper, S. (2003) 'The applied physiology and game analysis of rugby union'. *Sports Medicine*, 33: pp. 973-91

Epstein, Y., Rosenblum, R., Burstein, R. & Sawka, M. N. (1988) 'External load can alter energy cost of prolonged exercise'. *European Journal of Applied Physiology*, 57: pp. 243-7

Froelicher, V. F., Jr., Thompson, A. J., Jr., Noguera, I., Davis, G., Stewart, A. & Triebwasser, J. H. 'Prediction of maximal oxygen consumption: Comparison of the Bruce and Balke treadmill protocols'. *Chest*, 68: pp. 331-6

Hermansen, L. & Saltin, B. (1969) 'Oxygen uptake during maximal treadmill and bicycle exercise'. *Journal of Applied Physiology*, 26: pp. 31-7

Hill, J. & Timmis, A. (2002) 'ABC of clinical electrocardiography: Exercise tolerance testing. Clinical review'. *British Medical Journal*, 324: pp. 1084–7

Howley, E. T., Bassett, J. R. & Welch, H. G. (1995) 'Criteria for maximal oxygen uptake: Review and commentary'. *Medicine and Science in Sports and Exercise*, 27: pp. 1292-1301

Kline, G. M., Porcari, J. P., Hintermeister, R., Freedson, P. S., Ward, A., McCarron, R. F., Ross, J. & Rippe, J. M. (1987) 'Estimation of VO_2 max from a one-mile track walk, gender, age, and body weight'. *Medicine and Science in Sports and Exercise*, 19, pp. 253-9

Kyle, V. (1991) 'The 20-metre shuttle run test: A simple easy to administer aerobic fitness test'. *Sports Coach*, 15: pp. 6-7

Krustrup, P., Mohr, M., Amstrup, T., Rysgaard, T., Johansen, J., Steensberg, A., Pedersen, P. K. & Bangsbo, J. (2003) 'The Yo-Yo intermittent recovery test: Physiological response, reliability and validity'. *Medicine and Science in Sports and Exercise*, 35: pp. 697-705

Krustrup, P., Mohr, M., Nybo, L., Jensen, J. M., Nielsen, J. J. & Bangsbo, J. (2006) 'The Yo-Yo IR2 Test: Physiological response, reliability, and application to elite soccer'. *Medicine and Science in Sports and Exercise*, 38: pp. 1666-73

Laukkanen, R., Oja, P., Pasanen, M. & Vuori, I. (1992) 'Validity of a two-kilometre walking test for estimating maximal aerobic power in overweight adults'. *International Journal of Obesity and Related Metabolic Disorders*, 16: pp. 263-8

Leger, L. A., Mercier, D., Gadoury, C. & Lambert, J. (1988) 'The multistage 20 metre shuttle run test for aerobic fitness'. *Journal of Sports Sciences*, 6: pp. 93-101

Leger, L. A. & Lambert, J. (1982) 'A maximal multistage 20-m shuttle run test to predict VO_2 max'. *European Journal of Applied Physiology*, 49: pp. 1-12

Nicholas, C., Nuttall, F. & Williams, C. (2000) 'The Loughborough Intermittent Shuttle Test: A field test that simulates the activity pattern of soccer'. *Journal of Sports Sciences*, 18: pp. 97-104

Noakes, T., Myburgh, K. & Schall, R. (1990) 'Peak treadmill velocity during the VO_2 max test predicts running performance'. *Journal of Sports Sciences*, 8: pp. 35-45

Paliczka, V. J., Nichols, A. K. & Boreham, C. A. G. (1987) 'A multi-stage shuttle run as a predictor of running performance and maximal oxygen uptake in adults'. *British Journal of Sports Medicine*, 21: pp. 163-5

Ramsbottom, R., Brewer, J. & Williams, C. (1988) 'A progressive shuttle run test to estimate maximal oxygen uptake'. *British Journal of Sports Medicine*, 22: pp. 141-4

Shephard, R. J. (1984) 'Tests of maximum oxygen intake: A critical review'. *Sports Medicine*, 1: pp. 99-124

BLOOD LACTATE AND ANAEROBIC THRESHOLD TESTING

10

OBJECTIVES

After completing this chapter you should be able to:

1 Understand the concept of anaerobic threshold and the link between lactate and ventilatory threshold.
2 Appreciate the health and safety aspects of taking capillary blood samples from clients.
3 Realise the relationship between blood lactate and muscle lactate concentrations.
4 Estimate lactate threshold based on blood lactate measurements using different techniques.
5 Assess the efficacy of lactate threshold as a predictor of performance in sports or events.
6 Estimate ventilatory threshold based on gas analysis.
7 Explain the use of clinical measurement of anaerobic threshold, typically using ventilatory data.
8 Assess the environmental and nutritional factors that can affect results obtained from lactate testing.

Anaerobic threshold

As introduced in chapter 2, the energy systems of the body can generally be classified as either *aerobic* (with the use of oxygen) or *anaerobic* (without the use of oxygen), within which there are sub-classifications.

During a period of exercise, as the intensity increases, the proportion of energy delivered from anaerobic sources, to meet the demand, increases, while the proportion of energy from aerobic sources decreases.

Although many definitions of anaerobic threshold (AT) have been proposed over the years, Wasserman and colleagues in 1973 are commonly cited for stating it is *'the level of work or oxygen consumption at which metabolic acidosis and changes in gas exchange occur'*.

It was previously thought within the area of physiological scientific research that the human body produced lactate in response to a decrease in oxygen supply to the working muscles. It is now commonly agreed that this is not the case, as even fully oxygenated muscle fibres produce lactate when energy demands are high. The term anaerobic threshold is therefore somewhat misleading as the contribution of the anaerobic system to energy production is relatively minor during sub-maximal exercise. Some researchers now prefer to use the term *performance threshold* rather than anaerobic threshold.

The anaerobic threshold of an individual can be identified as a result of testing by using a range of both invasive and non-invasive methods such as the following:

Invasive methods

- Lactate threshold
- Onset of blood lactate accumulation (OBLA)
- Maximal lactate steady state (MLSS)
- Individual anaerobic threshold

Non-invasive methods

- Ventilatory threshold
- Anaerobic threshold

- First and second ventilatory threshold
- Heart rate deflection

These are just a small selection of some of the terms that are often used to refer to this transition between energy system contributions during increasing intensity exercise. To further confuse matters, various authors have differing definitions relating to the same threshold.

Despite these various differences, measurements (regardless of the testing method used) of anaerobic thresholds have a valuable role to play in both a sporting and a clinical environment.

It is generally agreed that there are four main reasons as to why measurements of anaerobic threshold are considered to be very useful as part of the physiological assessment of both athletic subjects and patients:

(1) Indicators of adaptations to training

While VO_2 max increases substantially with the onset of aerobic training in sedentary or untrained individuals, it is considered to be relatively stable and an insensitive marker of training in highly trained athletes. On the other hand, anaerobic threshold adapts by a much greater degree to training than VO_2 max (see figure 10.1). In this example the subject's VO_2 max was already high (as expected for an elite middle-distance runner) at $77ml^{-1}.kg^{-1}.min^{-1}$ and remained practically unchanged over this period. However, his anaerobic threshold (here indicated by OBLA) increased dramatically over this eight-week training block from 18 to 19km.h^{-1}. Therefore, in both recreationally active and well-trained individuals, anaerobic threshold is a more sensitive measure of responses to training than VO_2 max.

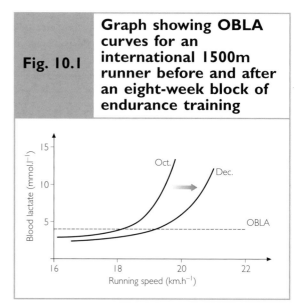

Fig. 10.1 Graph showing **OBLA** curves for an international 1500m runner before and after an eight-week block of endurance training

(2) Related to performance in endurance events

In addition to being a more sensitive measure of training than VO_2 max, anaerobic threshold is also considered to be a better predictor of endurance performance.

Anaerobic threshold is linked to the percentage of VO_2 max that can be sustained during prolonged endurance exercise, which plays a major role in determining exercise performance. Running speed or cycling power output at lactate threshold (LT) is also considered to be a very good predictor of endurance performance. For example, long-distance events such as a ten-mile run are often performed by athletes at an intensity that is close to the individual anaerobic threshold of that athlete.

NEED TO KNOW

Scientists supporting marathon world record holder, Paula Radcliffe, can predict her performance within a minute using laboratory-based physiological tests such as lactate threshold.

(3) Can be used to prescribe training intensities for athletes

Anecdotally, according to many endurance-based coaches, training at or around the anaerobic threshold represents a compromise, i.e. an intensity that is sufficiently high to produce significant aerobic training effects, but not so high as to induce fatigue too rapidly. This can ensure the optimum balance between intensity (speed) and volume (distance) for some of their training (threshold training).

It has been found that training at intensities around the lactate threshold seems to be effective in improving the lactate threshold in sedentary individuals but a higher intensity seems to be required for more highly trained endurance athletes.

(4) Can be used to prescribe exercise intensities and evaluate rehabilitation in clinical environments

In addition to testing athletes, assessment of anaerobic threshold testing also has a role to play with clinical patients. There is evidence that anaerobic threshold (typically assessed as ventilatory threshold) is reached before the ischemic threshold (the intensity at which coronary blood flow is compromised, resulting in inadequate oxygen delivery to the tissues).

Ischemic cardiovascular disease is the leading cause of death among adults in the developed world. It has been recommended by researchers such as Foster and colleagues in 2004 that patients with this disease exercise at an intensity of approximately 90 per cent of their individual ventilatory threshold to increase their fitness (which shouldn't risk further ischemia). Assessments of anaerobic threshold can also be used to assess cardiovascular functioning and thus how successfully the patient's rehabilitation is progressing.

Invasive measures of anaerobic threshold

Throughout research literature there are several terms used to define the intensity at which there is a dramatic increase in blood lactate concentration. Using these different definitions involves interpretation of curves and can result in a variety of intensities being defined as the lactate threshold, depending on the investigator. The assessment of the lactate threshold using the same set of lactate data can result in a range from 79 to 92 per cent of VO_2 max when using different techniques to interpret the data.

Lactate threshold testing typically involves repeated bouts of exercise at increasing workloads, completing between five and nine stages of increasing intensity. In typical testing protocols, increases in treadmill velocity range between 0.5 and 1.5km.h^{-1} for runners or between 20 and 50W for cyclists or rowers.

Jones protocol for heart rate response, lactate threshold, running economy and VO_2 max in runners

The British Association of Sport and Exercise Sciences (BASES) protocol for determining lactate threshold in middle- and long-distance runners has been developed by Andy Jones from the University of Exeter and is used by the English Institute of Sport (EIS).

This particular laboratory-based test is typically performed in two parts. The first part of the test is known as phase one and is used to determine several physiological parameters of the subject being tested.

Phase one testing

- running economy
- heart rate training zones
- lactate threshold

The second part of the test is known as phase two, which is then subsequently used to determine other physiological parameters of the same subject being tested.

Phase two testing

- VO_2 max
- peak heart rate

Required resources

Treadmill, heart rate monitor, stopwatch, lactate analyser, gas analyser.

General protocol

The main objective of the overall test is to complete between five and nine stages of exercise of progressively increasing intensity. The starting treadmill speed for this particular test is dependent on several factors (see table 10.1) such as the age and fitness of the subject.

Table 10.1	Starting speeds for different subjects
Type of athlete	Treadmill starting speed
Competitive junior male	13km.h^{-1}
Competitive junior female	11km.h^{-1}
An athlete who can run 6-min miles (16km.h^{-1}) for 10,000m/10-mile races	11 or 12km.h^{-1}
Elite male runners	14 or 15km.h^{-1}

Note: Treadmill gradient should be set at 1 per cent to compensate for the lack of wind resistance when running on a treadmill.

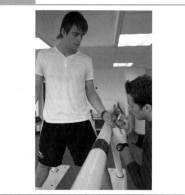

Fig. 10.2 A resting fingertip blood sample

Testing method

Phase one

1. Following a resting fingertip blood sample (see figure 10.2), subjects should perform a standardised 10 to 15-minute warm-up programme including stretching.
2. Subjects should exercise for three minutes at each stage and increase the treadmill velocity by 1km.h^{-1} for each subsequent stage.
3. Expired gases should be collected (see figure 10.3) for the final 50–60 seconds of each stage (accurately timed) and average heart rate should be recorded over the final 30 seconds of each stage.
4. At the end of each stage subjects should grab the guard rails, lift their legs and carefully stand with both feet astride the moving belt (as in figure 10.4). A capillary blood sample for determination of lactate concentration should be performed within the next 15–30 seconds.

Fig. 10.3	**Expired gas collection during the test**

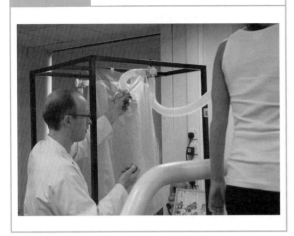

5. Subjects should then resume running at the increased treadmill speed, initially with their hands on the guard rails, partially supporting their weight (figure 10.4).

6. Phase one of testing should finish close to, but not at, exhaustion. Subjects should feel capable of completing one more stage if they were requested to. General criteria are a blood lactate concentration of above

Fig. 10.4	**End of stage position**

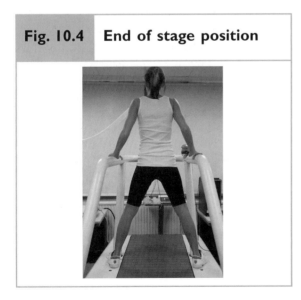

$4mmol.l^{-1}$ and heart rate within 5–10 beats of maximum.

Phase two

7. Subjects should then be allowed approximately 15 minutes of walking, jogging and stretching to recover before their final effort at phase two.

8. Starting treadmill speed for phase two should be the speed of the final stage reached on phase one, minus $2km.h^{-1}$. For example, if the subject finished at a speed of $19km.h^{-1}$ in phase one, start them at $17km.h^{-1}$ (and at a treadmill grade of 1 per cent) for the start of phase two.

9. Allow 1–2 minutes for the subject to reach this intensity and then commence timing. Increase the treadmill grade by 1 per cent every minute and expect subjects to last for between 5 and 10 minutes in total.

10. Collect expired gases from 4 per cent treadmill grade onwards (following the first three minutes) for the final 45 seconds of each stage.

11. If required, a post-exercise peak blood lactate sample could be obtained. Be aware that this should be taken immediately after exercise or at a fixed time-point post-exercise, for example five minutes.

Threshold points

During testing there appear to be two points or thresholds in blood lactate or ventilatory response to incremental exercise. Identification of where these thresholds occur, which requires a degree of interpretation, can be used in setting training intensities for the subject being tested.

With respect to lactate concentration, the first assumed point or threshold is considered to be the workload (exercise intensity) at which there is a significant increase in blood lactate concentration above resting level.

This first threshold is defined as the exercise intensity at which blood lactate concentration exceeds average resting values by 1mmol.l^{-1} (the term mmol.l^{-1} is the standard unit of concentration) and can be seen in figure 10.5 denoted by LT$_1$.

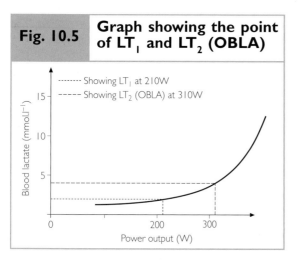

Fig. 10.5 Graph showing the point of LT$_1$ and LT$_2$ (OBLA)

The point during exercise at which threshold one typically occurs is approximately 2mmol.l^{-1}.

The second threshold is considered to be the point at which there is a very rapid, sustained increase in lactate concentration. The second threshold (denoted by LT$_2$ in figure 10.5) can be determined in several ways and typically occurs between 2.5 and 5.5mmol.l^{-1}. The second threshold often occurs at OBLA or MLSS, as described later in this chapter.

There are also graphical approaches to the determination of the point of threshold two. These approaches involve plotting lactate concentrations against workload/treadmill velocity during testing of an individual. One of the simplest and most commonly used methods of determination of lactate threshold is known as D$_{max}$. By using this method the threshold point can be obtained by drawing a straight line between the resting and peak exercise values of blood lactate concentration (see figure 10.6).

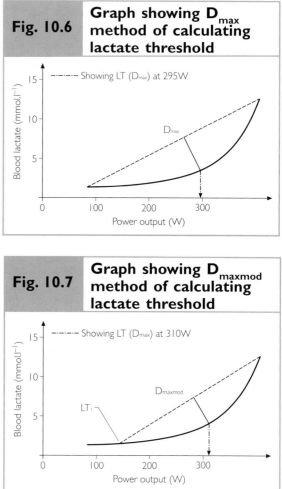

Fig. 10.6 Graph showing D$_{max}$ method of calculating lactate threshold

Fig. 10.7 Graph showing D$_{maxmod}$ method of calculating lactate threshold

The maximal distance between this line and the smoothed curve is referred to as D$_{max}$ and the exercise intensity equivalent to this point is assumed to be threshold two.

Another method used to determine threshold two is called ADAPT and was developed and is used by the Australian Institute of Sport (AIS). The same procedure as D$_{max}$ is used, but the starting point is not a resting exercise lactate as in D$_{max}$, but the threshold one point (see figure 10.7). This threshold point is called D$_{maxmod}$ and is higher than D$_{max}$.

Fixed blood lactate concentration (OBLA)

Some of the limitations of assessing thresholds have been discussed previously. As a result, many researchers advocate choosing a fixed blood lactate concentration to detect anaerobic threshold, as it is a more objective measure opposed to the more subjective interpretations of other methods. This fixed concentration was initially agreed among researchers to be $4.0mmol.l^{-1}$, but some investigators choose 2.0 or $2.4mmol.l^{-1}$. The workload equivalent to 2.0 or $2.5mmol.l^{-1}$ is often chosen as LT_1 (roughly equivalent to threshold one) and $4.0mmol.l^{-1}$ is chosen as LT_2 (also known as onset of blood lactate accumulation or OBLA) (see figure 10.5) and is equivalent to threshold two.

During lactate threshold testing, the duration of each exercise stage is normally set at 3–4 minutes. It is worth noting that an exercise intensity equivalent to a lactate concentration of $4.0mmol.l^{-1}$ reached at the end of a four-minute stage will typically be higher if the duration of exercise is longer than four minutes.

For the example illustrated in figure 10.5, if the cyclist exercised at 310W for 30–40 minutes, we would expect a higher blood lactate concentration of $5–6mmol.l^{-1}$, which indicates one of the limitations of using fixed blood lactate concentration methods. Another limitation is that a value of $4.0 mmol.l^{-1}$ is rather arbitrary, and will vary with the subject being tested. Also, the non-linear increase (known as an exponential increase) in blood lactate concentration may not occur at exactly $4.0mmol.l^{-1}$.

A major limitation of blood lactate testing is that the type of analyser used can affect the lactate concentration results obtained. For example, an exercise intensity equivalent to OBLA obtained from an Accusport portable lactate analyser may be $0.5–1.0km.h^{-1}$ lower than that obtained from the YSI1500 lactate analyser. The duration of each stage during testing will also affect the threshold results obtained. For example, longer stages (six minutes as opposed to three minutes as described in the protocol) will result in lower values for speed/power output being obtained.

In contrast, allowing longer recoveries between stages will result in higher values for speed/power output than shorter recoveries. The duration of stages and the recovery times between them are primarily dependent on the equipment and staff available for testing. Finally, using longer stages may provide more accurate values but may fatigue subjects prematurely, not allowing a true VO_2 max to be obtained in the second phase of testing as described in the Jones protocol above. Longer stages will also mean greater test durations and hence may limit the number of subjects that can be tested per day.

Maximal lactate steady state (MLSS)

It has long been established that low-intensity cardiovascular exercise results in an increase followed by a subsequent decrease in blood lactate concentration over time.

It has also been well documented that high-intensity cardiovascular exercise results in a continuous increase in blood lactate concentration over time.

It is assumed, therefore, that between these two exercise intensity states lies an exercise intensity level at which blood lactate will increase but then at some point will become stable (this is known as the steady state).

The highest exercise intensity level at which this steady state occurs is termed the *maximal lactate steady state* (MLSS). This can generally be determined by performing four to five repeated bouts of exercise of up to 30 minutes in duration at intensities of between 50 and 90 per cent of VO_2 max. MLSS values tend to be between 70 and 80 per cent of VO_2 max, slightly lower than the point of OBLA.

If, during a particular testing session, the subject's blood lactate concentration increases by more than 1.0mmol.l[-1] between 10 and 30 minutes of exercise, then it is not considered to be a steady state level and hence the MLSS would be deemed to have been exceeded.

MLSS testing in the laboratory is rather time-consuming, so a simpler approach sometimes used is to assess the lactate threshold of a subject during treadmill testing (as outlined previously) and then get the subject to exercise at that threshold intensity for 30 minutes (for example, a standard 'threshold' run). The lactate concentration at 10 and 30 minutes is measured and if it increases by more than 1.0mmol.l[-1] over that period then the intensity is considered to be above MLSS.

Example: using the example of a subject tested for the data shown in fig. 10.8, a threshold training intensity (18km.h[-1]) equivalent to a heart rate of 165bpm was established for training purposes. A week later the subject completed a 30-minute threshold run at 18km.h[-1]. Following testing, the subject's blood lactate concentration increased from 4.2 to 4.5mmol.l[-1] (between 10 and 30 minutes of exercise), indicating that the subject was very close to their individual maximal lactate steady state.

Fig. 10.8   Example subject data

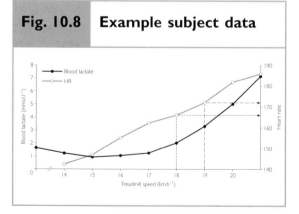

Another potential testing approach sometimes used is a method known as the *lactate minimum test* (LMT). This particular test allows for an estimation of MLSS from a single-test exercise session. This approach, however, is considered to be difficult to standardise and has not received universal approval.

Non-invasive anaerobic threshold markers

Ventilatory markers

As mentioned previously, lactate threshold is rarely used in clinical settings to determine an individual's anaerobic threshold. In these settings the ventilatory threshold (VT) is the parameter that is normally determined.

As with lactate thresholds, there are considered to be two thresholds for the ventilatory response to incremental exercise. These thresholds are known as VT_1 and VT_2. There is a consensus among many researchers that there is a link between ventilatory threshold (VT) and lactate threshold (LT).

Buffering of increasing quantities of lactate (by using sodium bicarbonate) in the blood results in increased (non-metabolic) CO_2 production. This excess CO_2 production stimulates an increase in ventilation beyond oxygen requirements and hence ventilatory threshold occurs.

NEED TO KNOW

Buffering is the term used to describe the ability of the body to regulate the acidity of the blood. In the case of exercise, hydrogen ions (charged particles) can increase the acidity of the blood and sodium bicarbonate tries to counteract this. Athletes often ingest large quantities of sodium bicarbonate in an attempt to improve this ability.

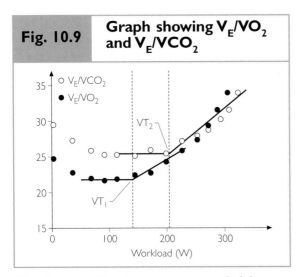

Fig. 10.9 Graph showing V_E/VO_2 and V_E/VCO_2

for carbon dioxide (V_E/VCO_2) (see figure 10.9). The point at which VT_1 occurs is approximately 50 per cent of VO_2 max and is equivalent to threshold one for blood lactates. The second threshold, VT_2, is normally identified as the point at which both V_E/VO_2 and V_E/VCO_2 increase (see figure 10.9). The point at which VT_2 occurs is approximately 85 per cent of VO_2 max, depending on the subject's fitness, and is equivalent to threshold two. These thresholds can be used to set training intensities. Typically, low intensity training would be lower than or equal to VT_1, moderate intensity would be between VT_1 and VT_2, and high intensity above VT_2.

This is not without controversy and debate as lactate threshold and ventilatory threshold are altered by manipulating the pedalling frequency in cyclists or by modifying the subject's muscle glycogen stores. Ventilatory threshold is greater than lactate threshold at 90rpm, but no different at 50rpm. In contrast, lactate threshold is greater than ventilatory threshold when a subject is glycogen depleted.

It has been demonstrated that neither blood lactate concentration nor acid levels increase in patients with MacArdle's disease, but ventilatory threshold still occurs.

Despite the controversies, ventilatory thresholds are useful and Spanish researcher Lucia and colleagues in 2004, using Tour de France cyclists, found that ventilatory threshold determined before the Tour was a good predictor of performance in time trials during the race.

There are many ways in which to assess these ventilatory thresholds VT_1 and VT_2. The first threshold, VT_1, can be determined as the point at which there is a non-linear increase in ventilation (V_E) and carbon dioxide production (VCO_2). This is determined as the point at which the ventilatory equivalent for oxygen (V_E/VO_2) increases without an increase in the ventilatory equivalent

Heart-rate deflection (Conconi test)

The Conconi test was developed in 1982 as a non-invasive method for estimating the anaerobic threshold. It is based on the linear relationship between heart rate and work rate (as running speed or power output increases, so does heart rate). There is a typical deflection from this relationship above a certain intensity, and some researchers have found a good relationship between this heart-rate deflection point and anaerobic threshold (Conconi and colleagues tend to be cited most). This is a controversial issue, however, as many researchers have found no such relationship.

One reason for this controversy is that no universally accepted explanation for why the deflection point occurs has been adopted. Those who support the use of heart-rate deflection propose that its occurrence is related to a slowdown in oxygen uptake with increasing exercise intensities.

Power outputs at anaerobic threshold estimated from heart-rate deflection testing are typically found to be between 13 and 28 per cent higher than those obtained from lactate threshold. Despite this criticism from the scientific community, heart-rate deflection is used by many coaches and athletes, as it is inexpensive and simple to implement. In this particular test the subject increases their speed gradually every 200 metres and the heart rate and time, at each 200-metre point, is recorded.

This gradual increase in speed every 200 metres is continued until the subject is unable to maintain the pace. The total distance covered by the test should be between 2.5 and 4km to ensure sufficient information is available for subsequent calculations. Speed versus heart rate is then plotted from which the subject's anaerobic threshold can be determined.

Required resources

Treadmill, heart rate monitor, stopwatch, pen and paper.

Testing method

1. The subject performs a 5 to 10-minute standardised warm-up programme.
2. Ensure that the heart rate of the subject is being recorded before the test commences.
3. Start the treadmill at the required starting speed.
4. Start the stopwatch and commence the test as the subject starts running.
5. Record the time and heart rate every 200 metres.
6. Increase the treadmill speed every 200 metres by 0.5km.hr^{-1}.
7. End the test when the subject has reached maximum heart rate or can no longer continue.
8. Stop the heart rate recording and timing.

Analysis

Plot the speed at every 200 metres against the heart rate on a graph such as that in figure 10.10. It is common that the graph is fairly straight to start with and then dips down before rising again. This dip in the graph is considered to

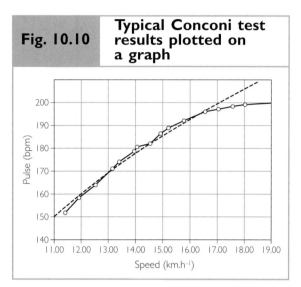

Fig. 10.10 Typical Conconi test results plotted on a graph

indicate the point of the subject's anaerobic threshold (occurring at approximately 14.5km/hr).

General test information

Anaerobic threshold test conditions

There are many factors that can affect the outcome of the results during lactate or threshold testing. The main factors include environment, muscle glycogen status and hydration levels of the subject being tested.

- The response of blood lactate to incremental testing can be affected by environmental factors. For instance, high ambient temperatures can increase blood lactate concentrations, resulting in lower than expected lactate thresholds being determined; thus when comparing values obtained in the laboratory and those obtained in a field environment, the differences in the testing temperatures should always be considered.
- Muscle glycogen is the main source of glucose for anaerobic glycolysis, resulting in lactate

production. It is likely that a subject's muscle glycogen may be depleted if they have exercised at a high intensity or for a long time and have not replaced the glycogen used by ingesting sufficient carbohydrate. If a subject starts a lactate threshold test with low muscle glycogen stores, lower lactate concentrations occur and hence lactate threshold may be overestimated. This is particularly a problem when fixed lactate concentrations are used, for example OBLA.

- Dehydration may result in elevated heart rate and if severe may also increase blood lactate concentrations, resulting in an underestimation of lactate thresholds.

For these main reasons (and other reasons not addressed in this book), it is important to ensure that all subjects to be tested are well rested from their last training session and that they have had a consistent diet sufficiently high in carbohydrates and fluids to prevent these potential problems from occurring. It is also important to try to standardise the testing environment as much as possible.

Interpreting test results

The effectiveness of training can be determined in middle-distance and endurance athletes based on blood lactate and ventilatory threshold responses.

Figure 10.11 illustrates a typical shift to the right at a given blood lactate concentration resulting from an increase in the subject's aerobic capacity. The shape of the curve and maximal blood lactate concentration remain similar, but the subject is working at higher blood lactate concentration. Figure 10.11 also illustrates a downward shift in the curve, resulting in lower blood lactate concentrations at a given exercise intensity, again a measure of lower production of lactate or an increased capacity for lactate

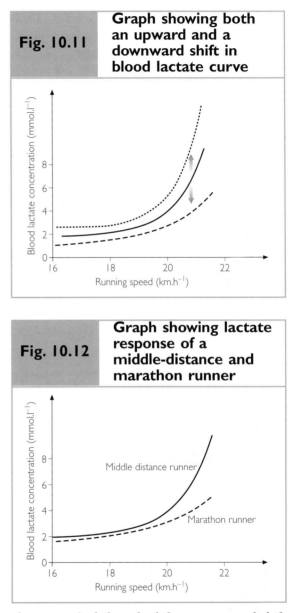

Fig. 10.11 Graph showing both an upward and a downward shift in blood lactate curve

Fig. 10.12 Graph showing lactate response of a middle-distance and marathon runner

clearance. A shift to the left or an upward shift indicates a decrease in aerobic capacity and may occur after a period of injury or detraining.

The difference in lactate response between athletes in different events can be reasonably pronounced. A middle-distance runner, for instance, tends to produce greater lactate concentrations, especially maximal lactate concentration, than athletes in more prolonged events such as marathons (see figure 10.12). This is thought to reflect the greater capacity for anaerobic metabolism in middle-distance athletes and greater capacity for aerobic metabolism in endurance athletes. Similar differences would be observed when comparing Olympic 3000-metre pursuit cyclists and cyclists competing in road events such as the Tour de France.

Ventilatory and lactate thresholds can also be used to set training intensities as outlined previously. Speed, workload or heart rate at each threshold can be used to set the intensity. One approach commonly used in endurance sports is outlined in table 10.2.

Table 10.2	Intensity levels for different types of training
Type of training	Intensity level
Easy or recovery	Below threshold 1
'Steady' or aerobic	Between threshold 1 and 2
'Threshold'	Equivalent to threshold 2
Interval or 'VO$_2$ max'	Above threshold 2

Laboratory-based and portable lactate analysers

The use of portable automated lactate analysers has dramatically increased the use of lactate testing in competitive sport. Years of development by manufacturers such as Boehringer Mannheim have increased the reliability and accuracy of lactate measurements. Boehringer Mannheim introduced the Accusport analyser in 1994 and it has been one of the most popular portable analysers used since then.

One of the limitations of portable lactate analysers, some of which are still used, is that the accuracy of the technique is dependent upon the volume of the blood sample. One of the Accusport's limitations is that it can be difficult to fix the volume of blood collected. This problem has been minimised with some handheld lactate analysers such as the Lactate Pro developed by Arkray KDK in Japan in 1997.

With these devices, the volumes collected (5μl) are more carefully controlled and hence closer to lactate values obtained from one of the gold standards for calibrating lactate concentration, the predominantly laboratory based YSI 1500.

Blood lactate concentrations obtained from

Fig. 10.13b	Portable lactate analysers

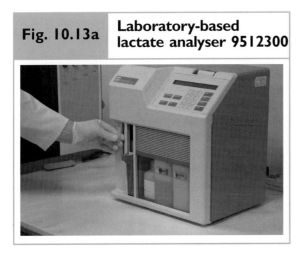

the Accusport tend to be higher than those obtained from the YSI 1500, whereas the authors have found that data from the Lactate Pro tends to be more accurate and reliable than the Accusport.

The choice of analyser is dictated by portability, set-up costs and personal preferences. It is clear, though, that lactate measurements collected using one type of analyser should not be compared to results obtained from another analyser.

The Lactate Pro costs approximately £200 plus £1.50 per sample analysed. The YSI 1500 is more accurate but less portable and requires greater technical knowledge and servicing. The YSI 1500 costs approximately £1500; the cost per sample is quite inexpensive compared to the Lactate Pro, but variable depending on how many samples are to be collected. For most coaches, a hand-held analyser such as the Lactate Pro would be a useful addition.

Lactate analysis is used predominantly in endurance sports but is becoming more prevalent in team sports and combat sports. For example, many English Premiership football teams perform lactate threshold testing on their first-team players.

Fig. 10.13a	Laboratory-based lactate analyser 9512300

Blood sampling techniques

Accurate methods of blood sampling are essential if the investigator requires reliable measurements of blood lactate concentration.

The sweat of an individual contains a greater concentration of lactate than blood; therefore, contaminating blood samples with sweat (or even alcohol) will result in highly variable and inaccurate results. More important than this accuracy of collection is the requirement to ensure that blood sampling is safe (for both the subject and the investigators) and minimises the infection risks.

Most blood sampling procedures in sports and event testing involve collection of:

• Arterial blood
• Venous blood
• Arterialised venous blood
• Capillary blood

Blood sampling via venepuncture

Arterial blood (blood from any artery in the body) is not routinely collected, due to the invasive nature of the process and the requirement for medically qualified staff. Venous blood

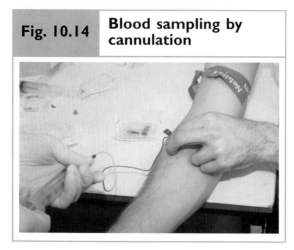

| Fig. 10.14 | Blood sampling by cannulation |

sampling (blood taken from a vein in the body) is performed when volumes of greater than 0.1ml are required.

For venous blood samples, a superficial (close to the surface of the body) forearm vein or ante-cubital (elbow) vein is typically chosen. If repeated samples are to be obtained, the subject may have a cannula attached (a device inserted into the vein or artery from which blood samples can be taken), which is kept from clotting by flushing after each blood sample with a small quantity of saline (salty water).

Reduce blood clotting by adding a very small quantity of heparin to the saline, though this process may require medical supervision.

In place of arterial blood, venous blood obtained from a heated superficial forearm vein is indistinguishable from arterial blood.

One 'rule of thumb' is that the person performing the blood sampling should make no more than three attempts to obtain a blood sample from the subject and after three failures, they should have another trained colleague replace them. Always record the number of blood samples and total blood volumes removed for each subject.

The small blood volumes typically obtained in sport science research are not normally large enough to stimulate erythropoesis (formation of new red blood cells), as there is a high risk of anaemia if large volumes of blood are removed from a repeatedly tested subject.

For venous blood sampling, in particular venous cannulation, medically qualified personnel or a trained phlebotomist is required. Those obtaining blood samples should be first-aid trained, as events such as patients fainting or going into shock, though rare, do occur. Blood sampling without consent could be considered as assault and, as mentioned earlier, informed consent must be obtained from subjects prior to testing.

Capillary blood sampling

The process of capillary blood sampling from the fingertip (figure 10.15a) or earlobe (figure 10.15b) is suitable for the collection of small quantities of blood of between 100 and 200μl.

Capillary blood sampling does not require the same degree of training or medical supervision as venepuncture and has lower health risks. Despite this, there is still a risk of infection and thus health and safety is still of concern.

The site of sample collection can affect the values obtained and depends on the nature of the sports/activities. For rowers or climbers, blood samples are commonly taken from the earlobe but in some testing on rowers the foot has been chosen, as it is relatively static during rowing ergometry. Sampling from the toe could possibly result in an increased risk of infection due to the area being normally covered. Fingertip sampling is not recommended for rowers or climbers, as the associated soreness may affect technique and contaminate the oar/climbing holds.

A recent study by Draper and colleagues in 2006 at the University of Chichester found that blood lactate concentrations were between 0.3 and 0.5mmol.l^{-1} greater from the fingertip than from earlobe samples. This is most likely due

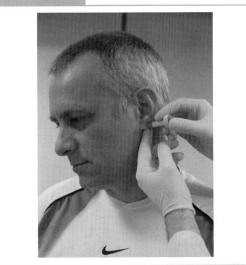

Fig. 10.15b   **Earlobe capillary sample**

to delays in the release of lactate into the central circulation resulting from localised changes in blood flow due to isometric contractions of the hands and forearms.

Similar results for lactate measurements from the toe have been found in rowers, with lactate values being similar between toe and earlobe, and lower than values obtained from fingertip samples.

For the fingertips, immersion of the hand in hot water (42°C) can arterialise the sample, producing a greater, and more free-flowing and reproducible, blood sample. For the earlobe, rubefacient cream such as Finalgon has the same effect. When sampling from earlobes, the cartilaginous area should not be punctured.

There are several choices for lancets, and new devices from Autoclic allow the disposed lancet to be kept within the device, and thus immediate access to a sharps container (bin used in laboratories to contain used sharp objects) for each sample is not required. With most lancets, the lancet depth may be altered to between 1 and 3mm, depending on the subject's skin thickness.

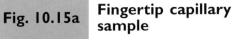

Fig. 10.15a   **Fingertip capillary sample**

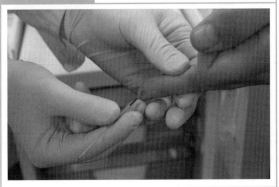

Fingertip capillary blood sampling for use with a Lactate Pro analyser

Required resources

Cotton wool pads or tissues, 70-per-cent alcohol pads, sterile lancets, hot water or rubefacient cream if required, sterile disposable gloves, sharps container and biohazard bag, Lactate Pro handset, Lactate Pro collection strips.

Testing method

1. Check calibration of analyser and initialise it for the collection strips you are going to be using, i.e. if the analyser is displaying F2, ensure that you are using F2 strips. Remove collection strip from packaging and insert into handset.
2. Ensure that you wash your hands with a liquid antimicrobial detergent and wear sterile, disposable gloves for each subject.
3. Select the sample site and warm the area if required.
4. Clean the site using an alcohol pad, starting in the centre and cleaning towards the periphery in a circular motion. Allow the alcohol to evaporate off and wipe the fingertip with a clean cotton pad.
5. The finger should be held firmly and the puncture should be made in one movement, perpendicular to the lines of the fingerprint and preferably not in the central, most sensitive area of the fingertip. This central area will often be calloused in rowers/climbers and should be avoided where possible.
6. The first drop of blood may be contaminated with sweat or alcohol and should be wiped away with a clean piece of cotton wool.
7. The finger should be 'milked' to encourage blood flow. Squeezing the site too vigorously may encourage blood flow, but will result in dilution of the sample with interstitial fluid and thus should be avoided.
8. (a) Introduce the Lactate Pro collection strip to the blood drop; it will take up 5µl by capillary action and 'beep' when this is complete. The lactate concentration will be displayed 60 seconds later. (b) If an analyser such as the YSI 2300 or YSI 1500 is to be used, the blood sample must be collected into an appropriate container, for example a capillary tube or specialised Eppendorf tube. One or two heparinised capillary tubes can be filled from a single puncture (100–200µl). Samples should be kept on ice to prevent clotting.
9. Provide the subject with some cotton wool to apply pressure to the sample site.
10. Dispose of all contaminated material into appropriate, clearly identified waste containers. Ensure that the lancets are disposed of into a sharps container, otherwise needle-stick injuries may occur. Ensure cleanliness of the blood sampling environment. Remove gloves and wash hands again using a liquid soap.

Storage and treatment of blood samples after collection

Whole blood is typically used for many analytical techniques to measure parameters such as blood glucose and lactate concentration. Since clotting occurs rapidly post collection, samples should be collected into tubes containing an anticoagulant such as potassium EDTA or heparin. If plasma is required, centrifugation of the whole blood is necessary. To obtain serum samples, whole blood should be left in a plain tube for at least one hour in a warm environment before centrifugation.

First aid, accidents and blood sampling

In most cases, blood sampling is uncomplicated but practitioners should be first-aid trained or have first-aid trained staff close at hand. One of the most common incidents is fainting. This occurs due to the subject's thoughts or sights of blood, or has even been known to be caused by the sound of the autolancet. Communicating with the subject during the blood sampling procedure can reassure them and help you gauge their degree of anxiety. When sampling from a standing subject, be aware of the risk of the subject falling over and be conscious of the safety of the surrounding environment. If a subject has fainted, remove any attached needles then move the subject to a supine position with feet slightly elevated. Following venepuncture, blood may leak into surrounding tissues, forming a haematoma (bruise). Remove the needle and apply pressure to the area for five minutes.

Further reading

Amann, M., Subudhi, A. W., Foster, C. (2004) 'Influence of testing protocol on ventilatory thresholds and cycling performance'. *Medicine and Science in Sports and Exercise*, 36: pp. 613-22

Amann, M., Subudhi, A. W. & Foster, C. (2006) 'Predictive validity of ventilatory and lactate thresholds for cycling time trial performance'. *Scandinavian Journal of Medicine and Science in Sports*, 16: pp. 27–34

Balke, B. (1963) 'A simple field test for the assessment of physical fitness'. *Civil Aeromedical Research Institute Report*, 63: pp. 1-8

Ballarin, E., Sudhues, U., Borsetto, C., Casoni, J., Grazzi, G., Guglielmi, C., Manfredinin, F., Mazzoni, G. & Conconi, F. (1996) 'Reproducibility of the Conconi Test: Test repeatability and observer variations'. *International Journal of Sports Medicine*, 17: pp. 520-4

Bassett, D. R. & Howley, E. T. (2000) 'Limiting factors for maximum oxygen uptake and determinants of endurance performance'. *Medicine and Science in Sports and Exercise*, 32: pp. 70-84

Beaver, W. L., Wasserman, K. & Whipp, B. J. (1986) 'A new method for detecting anaerobic threshold by gas exchange'. *Journal of Applied Physiology*, 60: pp. 2020-7

Berg, K. (2003) 'Endurance training and performance in runners: Research limitations and unanswered questions'. *Sports Medicine*, 33: pp. 59-73

Bishop, D. (2001) 'Evaluation of the Accusport Lactate Analyser'. *International Journal of Sports Medicine*, 22: pp. 525-30

Bodner, M. & Rhodes, E. (2000) 'A review of the concept of the heart rate deflection point'. *Sports Medicine*, 30: pp. 31-46

Bosquet, L., Leger, L. & Legros, P. (2002) 'Methods to determine aerobic endurance'. *Sports Medicine*, 32: pp. 675-700

Conconi, F., Ferrari, M., Ziglio, P., Droghetti, P. & Codeca, L. (1982) 'Determination of the anaerobic threshold by a noninvasive field test in runners'. *Journal of Applied Physiology: Respiratory, Environmental and Exercise Physiology*, 52: pp. 869-73

Conconi, F., Grazzi, G., Casoni, I., Guglielmi, C., Borsetto, C., Ballari, N. E., Mazzonin, G., Patracchini, M. & Manfredinin, F. (1996) 'The Conconi test: Methodology after 12 years of application'. *International Journal of Sports Medicine*, 17: pp. 509-19

Davis, J. A. (1985) 'Anaerobic threshold: Review of the concept and directions for future research'. *Medicine and Science in Sports and Exercise*, 17: pp. 6-18

Draper, N., Brent, S., Hale, B. & Coleman, B. (2006) 'The influence of sampling site and assay method on lactate concentration in response to rock climbing'. *European Journal of Applied Physiology*, 98: pp. 363-72

Edwards, A. M., Clark, N. & MacFayden, A. M. (2003) 'Lactate and ventilatory thresholds reflect the training status of professional soccer players where maximum aerobic power is unchanged'. *Journal of Sports Science and Medicine*, 2: pp. 23-29

Forsyth, J. J. & Farrally, M. R. (2000) 'A comparison of lactate concentration in plasma collected from the toe, ear, and fingertip after a simulated rowing exercise'. *British Journal of Sports Medicine*, 34: pp. 35-8

Faria, E. W., Parker D. L. & Faria, I. E. (2005) 'The science of cycling: Physiology and training – part 1'. *Sports Medicine*, 35: pp. 285-312

Fell, J. W., Rayfield, J. M., Gulbin, J. P. & Gaffney, P. T. (1998) 'Evaluation of the Accusport Lactate Analyser'. *International Journal of Sports Medicine*, 19: pp. 199-204

Grazzi, G., Casoni, I., Mazzoni, G., Uliari, S. & Conconi, F. (2005) 'Protocol for the Conconi test and determination of the heartrate deflection point'. *Physiological Research*, 54: pp. 473-5

Jones, A. M. (2007) 'Middle- and long-distance running'. In Winter, E. M., Jones, A. M., Davison, R. C., Bromley, P. & Mercer, T. (eds.) *Sport and Exercise Science Testing Guidelines: The British Association of Sport and Exercise Sciences Guide. Volume I: Sport Testing*, London and New York: Routledge, pp. 147-56.

Jones, A. M. & Doust, J. (1995) 'The relationship of lactate minimum velocity to 8km running performance and comparison with other methods of determining 'aerobic threshold'. *Journal of Sports Sciences*, 13: p. 34

Jones, A. M. & Doust, J. (1997) 'The Conconi test is not valid for estimation of the lactate turnpoint in runners'. *Journal of Applied Physiology*, 15: pp. 385-94

Kubukeli, Z. N., Noakes, T. D. & Dennis, S. C. (2002) 'Training techniques to improve endurance exercise performances'. *Sports Medicine*, 32: pp. 489–509

Lucia, A., Hoyos, J., Perez, M., Santalla, A., Earnest, C. P. & Chicharro, J. L. (2004) 'Which laboratory variable is related to time trial performance in the Tour de France?' *British Journal of Sports Medicine*, 38: pp. 636-40

Maughan, J. B., R., Shirreffs, J. B. & Leiper, (2007) 'Blood sampling'. In Winter, E. M., Jones, A. M., Davison, R. C., Bromley, P. & Mercer, T. (eds.) *Sport and Exercise Science Testing Guidelines: The British Association of Sport and Exercise Sciences Guide. Volume I: Sport Testing*, London and New York: Routledge, pp. 25-9

McNaughton, L. R., Thompson, D., Philips, G., Backx, K. & Crickmore, L. (2002) 'A comparison of the Lactate Pro, Accusport, Analox GM7 and Kodak Ektachem Lactate Analysers in normal, hot and humid conditions'. *International Journal of Sports Medicine*, 23: pp. 130-5

Ozcelik, O. & Kelestimur, H. (2004) 'Effects of acute hypoxia on the determination of anaerobic threshold using the heart rate–work rate relationships during incremental exercise tests'. *Physiological Research*, 53: pp. 45-51

Saunders, A. C., Feldman, H. A., Correia, C. E. & Weinstein, D. A. (2005) 'Clinical evaluation of a portable lactate meter in type I glycogen storage disease'. *Journal of Inherited Metabolic Diseases*, 28: pp. 695-701

Sjodin, B. & Jacobs, I. (1981) 'Onset of blood lactate accumulation and marathon running performance'. *International Journal of Sports Medicine*, 2: pp. 23-26

Viru, A. & Viru, M. (2001) *Biochemical Monitoring of Sports Training*, Champaign, Illinois: Human Kinetics

Wasserman, K., Whipp, B. J., Koyal, S. & Beaver, W. L. (1973) 'Anaerobic threshold and respiratory gas exchange during exercise'. *Journal of Applied Physiology*, 35: pp. 236-43

Glossary

Acceleration   The rate of change of velocity

Acetylcholine (Ach)   Neurotransmitter substance released from several types of neurones

Acetyl coenzyme A   Produced from the breakdown of pyruvic acid

Actin   Protein structure within a muscle cell

Adaptation   Change due to repeated stimuli such as resistance training

Adenosine triphosphate (**ATP**)   Main energy currency of the cell

Adenosine diphosphate (**ADP**)   ATP with one phosphate group missing

Adenosine monophosphate (**AMP**)   ATP with two phosphate groups missing

Adrenal medulla   An endocrine gland that releases adrenaline and noradrenaline

Aerobic   In the presence of oxygen

Aerobic fitness   The ability to deliver oxygen to the working muscles and use it during exercise

Afferent nerves   Nerves that carry electrical signals from muscles to the central nervous system

Agility   A rapid whole-body movement with change of velocity or direction in response to a stimulus

Agonist   Refers to a muscle or muscle group responsible for the main action

Air-displacement plethysmography   Direct method of assessing body composition

Alveoli   Air sac in the lungs

Anaerobic   In the absence of oxygen

Anaerobic capacity   The total amount of energy that can be produced anaerobically during a bout of exercise

Anaerobic fitness   The ability to perform maximal intensity exercise

Anaerobic glycolysis   The breakdown of glucose (or glycogen) in anaerobic conditions (without the presence of oxygen)

Anaerobic power   The maximal rate at which energy can be produced

Anaerobic threshold   The point at which the energy demand of the exercise being carried out can no longer be met by the aerobic system

Android   Distribution of fat around the middle of the body

Anhydrous   Has no water in it

Antagonist   Refers to a muscle or muscle group responsible for opposing the main action

Anthropometry   The science relating to the measurement of body mass and proportions of the human body

Aorta   The main artery leading away from the left ventricle

Arrhythmia   Deviation from normal heartbeat

Asthma   Type of obstructive lung disease

Atherosclerosis   Narrowing and hardening of the arteries

Atrial fibrillation   Disorganised contraction of the atria resulting in ineffective pumping of blood to the ventricle

Atrium   Chamber in the heart which receives blood from blood vessels

Avascular   Lack of blood supply

Axon   Branch of a motor neuron

Baroreceptor   Pressure receptor that is sensitive to stretching as a result of pressure changes

Beta oxidation   Process of producing acetyl co-enzyme A within the aerobic energy system

Bio-electrical impedance   Indirect method of assessing body composition

Blood pressure   The force of the blood on the artery walls

BMI   Body mass index

Bradycardia   Low resting heart rate

Broncho-constriction   Type of obstructive lung disease

Calorie   The amount of energy needed to increase the temperature of 1g of water by 1°C

Capillary   The smallest type of blood vessel

Cardiac cycle   The sequence of contraction and relaxation of the heart

Cardiac output   The amount of blood pumped out of each ventricle per minute

Cardiovascular disease   Disease of the heart (and related vessels)

Centre of gravity   The point at which the body can be balanced

Cholesterol   A fat-like steroid used to form cell membranes

Co-contraction   Tension developed in an agonist and antagonist muscle

Collagen   The protein substance of connective tissue

Concentric contraction   A muscular contraction against a resistance in which the muscle length shortens

Contraction   Electrical stimulation of muscle to shorten

Correlation   The relationship between two measurements or groups of measurements

Criterion measure   The most valid testing method for a particular characteristic

Dehydration   Water loss from a state of normal amounts of body water

Delayed onset muscle soreness   Perception of post-exercise soreness

Densitrometry   Direct method of assessing body composition

Developmental stretch   A stretch held long enough to induce physical structure development to increase flexibility

Diaphragm   Muscle used for breathing

Diastolic   The time between the ventricle contractions when it is filling

Dyslipidemia   Abnormal amount of lipids in the blood

Eccentric contraction   A muscular contraction against a resistance in which the muscle lengthens

EIA   Exercise induced asthma

EIB   Exercise induced bronchoconstriction

Elasticity   The ability to resist deformation and return to the original shape

Electrocardiogram (ECG)   Device used to record the electrical activity of the heart

Electron transport chain   Part of an energy system pathway used in the production of ATP

Emphysema   Destruction of the surface of the alveoli

Energy   The capacity to do work

Endocrine system   An integrated system of organs, glands and tissues that involve the release of extracellular signalling molecules known as hormones

Energy system   A term used to describe the source or pathway of producing ATP

Enzymes   Proteins that can speed up chemical reactions

EPOC   Excess post-exercise energy consumption   The total oxygen consumed after exercise (of whatever intensity) in excess of a pre-exercise baseline level

Erythrocyte   A red blood cell

Expired air   Air that is breathed out

Extension   Movement at a joint in which the joint angle increases

External rotation   Rotation of a part of the body away from the mid-point

F = ma   Newton's law of acceleration

Fast twitch   Type of muscle fibre associated with strength and speed

Fatigue index   The percentage decrease in power from peak to minimal power output

Flexibility   The available range of motion around a specific joint

Flexion   Movement at a joint in which the joint angle decreases

Force   The weight of an object multiplied by 9 81

Forced expiratory ratio   The ratio between FVC and FEV_1

Forced expiratory volume in 1 second   The volume of air exhaled during the first second of forced expiration

Forced vital capacity   The volume of air exhaled during a forced maximal exhalation following a forced maximal inhalation

Golgi tendon organs   Proprioceptors in tendons sensing force and stretch

Goniometry   Measurement of joint angles

Gravity   Force of attraction caused by the earth

Haemoglobin   Part of a red blood cell that carries oxygen or carbon dioxide

Gynoid   Distribution of fat around the hips and thighs

Heart rate   The number of heart beats per minute (bpm)

High-density lipoprotein   Cholesterol transporters often referred to as the 'good cholesterol' by transporting cholesterol to the liver to be broken down and excreted

Histamine   A chemical in the body that has the effect of narrowing the airways

Hormone   A chemical messenger in the body

Hyperglycaemia   High levels of blood glucose

Hyperplasia   An increase in the number of muscle fibres

Hypertension   High blood pressure

Hypertrophy   Enlargement of an organ such as muscle

Hypocapnia   Very low pressure of carbon dioxide in the blood

Hypotension   Low blood pressure

Inspired air   Air that is breathed in

Insulin   A hormone secreted by the pancreas, which reduces blood sugar levels

Intensity   A measurement of the difficulty level or 'hardness' of the exercise

Internal rotation   Rotation of a part of the body towards the mid-point

Ion   A positively or negatively charged particle

Ischemia   A low oxygen state (normally due to blocked arteries)

Isoinertial contraction   Another term for isotonic

Isokinetic contraction   Muscle contraction where the joint angle speed is constant

Isometric contraction   Muscle contraction where there is no change in the muscle length

Isotonic contraction   Muscle contraction against a constant load as in free-weight training

Kinesiology   Study of the causes and effects of human movement

Korotkoff sound   Knocking sound associated with blood pressure measurements

Krebs cycle (TCA)   Part of an energy system pathway used in the production of ATP

Lactic acid   A waste product as a result of glycogen breakdown without the presence of oxygen

Leukocyte   White blood cell

Ligament   Tissue in the body that connects bone to bone used for support

Lipid   The overall term used to describe any fat-soluble molecule

Lipolysis   Breakdown of triglyceride to fatty acids and glycerol

Low-density lipoprotein   Known as the 'bad cholesterol' Tends to deposit cholesterol on blood vessel walls

MAOD   Maximal accumulated oxygen deficit A measurement of the oxygen deficit obtained by an individual during exhaustive maximal exercise

Mass   The quantity of matter a body contains

Mast cell   Place in the body from which histamines are released

Maximum heart rate (MHR)   Theoretically the maximum possible heart rate for an individual

Mechanical efficiency   The amount of energy required to perform a task in relation to the actual work accomplished Often referred to as Running Economy (RE)

Mean   The mean or arithmetic average is the sum of the scores divided by the number of scores

Median   The middle score or 50th percentile Order the numbers from low to high and the middle one is the median

Metabolic equivalent   A method of expressing energy expenditure

Metabolic syndrome   A combination of abdominal obesity, hypertension, dyslipidemia and impaired fasting glucose

Millimetres   A small unit of distance

Mitochondria   The 'power cell' or site of aerobic energy production

MMV   Maximum minute ventilation

Mode   The most frequently observed score Not typically a useful indicator of the average value for a measurement.

Motoneurone   Nerves that transmit signals away from the central nervous system to the muscles

Muscle spindle   Structures within muscle that detect changes in length

Muscular endurance   The ability of a muscle or muscle group to perform repeated contractions against a resistance over a period of time

Muscular strength   The maximum amount of force a muscle or muscle group can generate

MVC   Maximum Voluntary Contraction

MVV   Maximum Voluntary Ventilation

Myocardial Infarction   Irreversible injury to the heart muscle

Myocardium   Essentially the heart muscle

Myofibril   The smallest muscle fibre

Myosin   Protein structure within a muscle cell

Neural   Relating to the nervous system

Neuromuscular   Relating to the muscular and associated nervous system

Noradrenaline   A stress hormone

Obesity   The percentage body fat at which the risk of disease to the individual is increased

Objectivity (test)   The degree to which multiple scorers or testers agree on the magnitude and outcome of the score or measurement being taken

Origin   The attachment point of a muscle to a bone nearest to the midline of the body

Osteoporosis   A condition of reduced bone density

Oxygen deficit   The difference between the required oxygen volume and the volume actually used during a period of exercise

Palpation   The part of a physical examination in which an object or subject is felt

Parasympathetic nervous system   Division of the autonomic nervous system that can slow the heart rate

PAR-Q   Physical Activity Readiness Questionnaire   A common health screening questionnaire.

PEFR   Peak expiratory flow rate

Perceived exertion   A subjective measurement of exercise intensity

Phospho-creatine (PCr)   A chemical compound stored in the muscles

Phosphofructokinase (PFK)   A key enzyme used in glycolysis

Plasma   Major fluid component of blood in which blood cells are suspended

Plyometric   Rapid eccentric loading followed by a brief isometric phase and explosive rebound using stored elastic energy and powerful concentric contractions

Power   The product of force and velocity Power = Work (force x distance) ÷ Time

Prone   Lying on the front

Proprioception   Sense of position in space

Proprioceptive neuromuscular facilitation This is a type of partner-assisted stretching

Proximal   The segment of the body closest to the centre of the body

Pyruvate   Formed as a stage in the breakdown of glucose

Range   The range is the maximum score minus the minimum score It gives a measure of the variability of the data

Reciprocal inhibition The term used to describe the amount of relaxation elicited in the antagonist muscle when the agonist muscle contracts

Residual volume The volume of gas remaining in the lungs at the end of a maximal expiration

Resting heart rate (RHR) The heart rate at resting levels measured in beats per minute (bpm)

RM Repetition maximum

Sarcomere Unit of contraction in skeletal muscle

Screening A process used to determine health status

Sensitivity (test) The degree to which the measures taken reflect an improvement

Sigma A Greek symbol used to denote standard deviation

Sino atrial node The impulse-generating 'pacemaker' located in the right atrium

Skill Proficiency at a particular task

Skin folds Indirect method of assessing body composition

Slow twitch Type of muscle fibre associated with endurance

SO fibres Slow oxidative muscle fibres that require oxygen to produce contraction

Smooth muscle Muscle found in the walls of hollow organs that is not under voluntary control

Speed Movement per unit time with no particular direction

Sphygmomanometer A device that operates on barometric pressure in a mercury element used to measure blood pressure

Spirometer Device used for testing lung function

SPSS Statistical analysis package for social sciences

Stability A body's resistance to the disturbance of equilibrium

Stadiometer Device used to measure height

Standard deviation A statistic that shows how the data points are clustered around the mean (average) in a set of data

Stretching The method or technique used to influence the joint range of motion

Stretch reflex Reflex action causing contraction within a muscle

Stride length Distance covered ÷ Number of strides

Stride frequency Number of strides ÷ Time taken

Stroke volume The amount of blood ejected from one ventricle per heartbeat

Supine Lying on the back

Sympathetic nervous system Division of the autonomic nervous system, which can speed up the heart rate

Synergist A muscle or muscle group responsible for assisting the action

Systolic Maximum pressure on the artery walls during contraction of the left ventricle

Tachycardia High resting heart rate

Telemetry Method of remotely checking heart rate

Tendon Connective tissue that surrounds muscle fibres

Tidal volume The volume of air that is inhaled or exhaled with each breath

Tissue A collection of cells with a physiological function

TLC Total lung capacity

Transversus abdominis Muscle of the core involved in forced expiration

Triglyceride Type of fat used for fuel in the body

T-test Used to test the means of two normally distributed populations

Validity (test) Purported to specifically measure what the tester or testing team is investigating

Vasoconstriction Narrowing of the lumen of blood vessels

Vasodilation Increase in size of lumen of blood vessels

Vein A vessel that carries blood back to the heart

Velocity Movement per unit time with direction

Ventricle A chamber in the heart that receives blood from the atrium

Vestibular Balance information sent to the brain as a result of the mechanism of the inner ear

Voluntary As a result of conscious thought

VO$_2$ Symbol for oxygen consumption

VO$_2$max Symbol for maximal oxygen consumption, the maximum amount of oxygen that can be delivered to and consumed by the working muscles

Watts A unit of power

WHO World Health Organisation

WHR Waist to hip ratio

Work Force x Distance ÷ Time

Index

Notes

ALSO AVAILABLE IN THE *FITNESS PROFESSIONALS* SERIES

The Advanced Fitness Instructor's Handbook by Morc Coulson and David Archer

The Advanced Fitness Instructor's Handbook follows on from *The Fitness Instructor's Handbook*. It is the first textbook to cover the National Occupational Standards and the Qualifications framework for Level 3 and Level 4 Instructors teaching Exercise and Fitness – required to teach one-on-one, and the standards which gyms are increasingly expecting staff to attain. Includes photos and illustrations throughout.

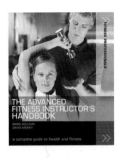

The Fitness Instructor's Handbook by Morc Coulson

The Fitness Instructor's Handbook is the essential guide for anyone working in, or wishing to enter, the fitness industry. It covers every component of the industry standards for both Level 2 and 3 qualifications, and offers the perfect blend of theory and practice on every aspect of health and fitness. Subjects include: the skeletal system; muscles and tendons; the energy system; circulation and respiration; screening clients; planning your own fitness programme and health and safety. Illustrated throughout by photos and illustrations.

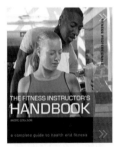

The Personal Trainer's Handbook by Rebecca Weissbort

The Personal Trainer's Handbook is a one-stop practical reference guide to the day-to-day running of a personal training business, covering: essential business skills; personal development; how to deal with clients and reference material, including sample forms that the reader can use, useful websites and professional bodies.

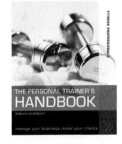

Available from all good bookshops or online. For more details on these and other A&C Black sport and fitness titles, please go to www.acblack.com.

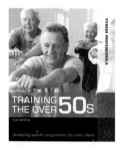

Training the Over 50s by Sue Griffin

This is the definitive handbook for any fitness professional who works with older adults. The 50-plus age range is one of the fastest growing groups of regular gym goers and they are increasingly turning to personal trainers and fitness instructors for guidance. Includes: the relationship between fitness and ageing; training adults with chronic conditions and designing individual programmes.

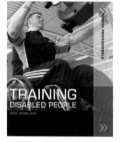

Training Disabled People by Sara Wicebloom

This is the only book to provide fitness professionals with detailed guidance on working with disabled clients. Written to the National Standards, it includes information on: medical conditions and how to research them; programming and instruction skills; pre-exercise checks and fitness testing; communication skills (including sign language); motivation techniques and sample programmes and exercises, fully illustrated with B&W photography.

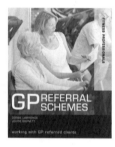

GP Referral Schemes by Debbie Lawrence & Louise Barnett

Exercise can help improve a wide variety of health problems, including obesity, heart disease, depression and mobility disorders, and GPs are increasingly referring their patients to local fitness professionals as part of their treatment. This book gives fitness professionals everything they need to know to manage a referred client, from fulfilling government recommendations to motivating and retaining clients, and includes: an outline of government policy; exercise guidelines for different medical conditions; designing a programme; sample client evaluation and assessment questionnaires and client starter packs.

Available from all good bookshops or online. For more details on these and other A&C Black sport and fitness titles, please go to www.acblack.com.